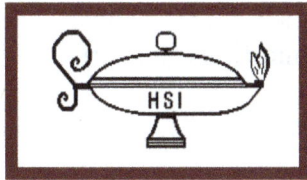

Conceptual Design Standards
for a
SINGLE COMPREHENSIVE HEALTH RECORD DATABASE COMMUNICATIONS NETWORK

AS RESEARCHED
by
HEALTH SYSTEMS INSTITUTE INC.

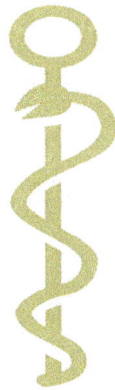

by
John R. Krismer - MHA-LFACHE
Principle Investigator

CCB Publishing
British Columbia, Canada

Conceptual Design Standards for a Single Comprehensive
Health Record Database Communications Network

Copyright ©2017 by John R. Krismer
ISBN-13   978-1-77143-300-6
First Edition

Library and Archives Canada Cataloguing in Publication
Krismer, John R., 1927-, author
Conceptual Design Standards for a Single Comprehensive Health Record
Database Communications Network / by John R. Krismer – First edition.
Issued in print and electronic formats.
ISBN 978-1-77143-300-6 (pbk.).--ISBN 978-1-77143-301-3 (pdf)
Additional cataloguing data available from Library and Archives Canada

Publisher: CCB Publishing
              British Columbia, Canada
              www.ccbpublishing.com

DEDICATION

A special thank you to my wife, Betty, and my children, Mike, Lynn, Stephen, Debbie, and Patty who always supported my work, helping me maintain a professional mission in health care. They supported my writing this book, so that others might benefit by my research, knowing that it might further stimulate quality health care professionals to continue their search for excellence.

ACKNOWLEDGMENTS

To those healthcare professionals who volunteered their time in developing the HSI standards. To Dr. Ian Brown, who persuaded the author to do research; To Dr. Hilliard Jason, who helped establish the Michigan State Medical School and supported the HSI concept, and the development of the paperless health record; To Bill Wallace, gold medal winner of the American College of Health Care Executives, who persuaded me to establish Health Systems Institute (HSI); To Bill Norris, past President of Control Data Corporation, who supported my research and developed the Digiscribe at no cost to HSI; To James Hamilton, the former director of the University of Minnesota Graduate Program in Hospital Administration and the past President of Hamilton Associates, who supported and promoted the HSI concept; To Dr. Lawrence Weed, who promoted the health record database concept and HSI, and authored the *Problem-Oriented Medical Record*; To Linda Pfeffer and Pat Larsen, past Presidents of the American Medical Records Administrators, who both worked with HSI committees in the design of the paperless medical record; To Drs. Jerry Cordez, and Bob Stow and all their associates, who coordinated the physicians of Lansing; To Donna Deary and Judy Waskeweitz and all their nursing associates, who helped define the nursing observations; To Dean Mc Creary, M.D., former head of the British Columbia Medical School, and Lloyd Detwiller, former President of the University of British Columbia hospitals. To Doctor Bill Knisely, the head of Michigan States Medical School who supported the HSI research; To Sister Albert Marie, former President of St. Lawrence Hospital, and Sister Mary Carroll, past Provincialate of the Sisters of St. Francis.

Contents

A BRIEF HISTORY OF
HEALTHCARE IN THE 20ᵗʰ CENTURY

Blue Cross was founded in 1929, and Blue Shield in 1939 with Blue Cross providing coverage for hospital services and Blue Shield covering physicians' services under this privately owned non-profit-noninsurance program that paid no taxes and was regulated by each state. Community rating was the Blue's trademark, which meant that everyone paid the same rate for their healthcare regardless of age, sex, where they lived, or how sick they were — making equal quality healthcare available to every consumer that purchased the Blue's healthcare coverage. The Blues paid a fair and equitable price for hospital services, facilities, equipment, and products and also paid doctors reasonable fees for the practice of medicine — back when U.S. healthcare was ranked number one in the world as this outstanding program became so successful it rapidly expanded to Canada, Puerto Rico, and Jamaica. The American Hospital Association (AHA) adopted the Blue Cross symbol in 1939 as the non-profit healthcare plan that was the only plan available and it provided excellent healthcare protection under a state regulated single prepayment program for some 106 million Americans. In the 1960's, the government also chose to partner with Blue Cross and Blue Shield (BCBS) to administer Medicare services. However this all began to change when commercial profit insurance companies lobbied their way into being approved by Congress to provide healthcare insurance and compete with the Blues. The McCarran–Ferguson Act, 15 U.S.C. §§ 1011-1015, known as Public Law 15, was passed on March 9, 1945, which became a United States federal law that exempted all profit insurance companies from most federal regulation, including a limited number of federal antitrust laws. This *Act* allowed profit insurance to lobby Congressmen for favors and not one Congressman stepped forward to protect the consumer's remarkable Community Rated Blues plan. Healthy younger individuals and working groups were persuaded to buy cheaper tiered low-risk "Group Rated" profit insurance policies from totally unregulated profit seeking insurance companies — not understanding that each group rate would significantly increase as its members decreased in number due to an increase in health related problems and age. The consumer was also completely unaware that the states and the federal government had no control over the spiraling healthcare costs that resulted from this unwise decision to make a profit from this country's sick and disabled. As a result, the Blues were increasingly forced to cover more and more of the sick and indigent and the female pregnancies, which the commercial companies dumped by increasing their premiums to unrealistic levels. The uncontrolled insurance donations to Congress also opened the door to funding many members of Congress in their re-election campaigns as they openly accepted these financial gifts for corporate favors. Today, we as a nation have a far better understanding of the dangerous underlying strategy that prompted our Congress to pass the McCarran-Ferguson Act — and why the Blues became so frustrated by the lack of public support. What it also tells us, is that Congress really didn't care about protecting the people's once very successful non-profit healthcare system, which was then ranked first in the world by the World Health Organization (WHO), rather than 32nd as we're ranked today. It's hard to believe that these are the same politicians that also once supported the Hill Burton U.S. federal law that provided federal tax dollar grants to guarantee hospital loans to improve this nation's growing healthcare facility needs after two world wars. This Hill Burton Act is what allowed the states to achieve a 4.5 beds per 1,000 population ratio — and these facilities were not allowed to discriminate based on race, color, national origin, or creed. Because profit insurance now has us well on our way to the total destruction of our once very efficient comprehensive human healthcare service to mankind, we need to also be very cautious of any destruction of our educational system as well as the infrastructure development of our highways and bridges that were once very cost effective tax supported community services. Yes, profits are soaring for the very wealthy corporations and our Congressmen who have suddenly become the benefactors, rather than the sick and indigent of this great country. So although we now live in the richest country in the history of this world, in reality it means very little to the general population because almost all of today's wealth is controlled by only a few of the very powerful and closely connected large corporations. Looking back to the 1960's, we now find there has been an enormous transfer of trillions of dollars from the middle class and the poor to the wealthy, thereby exposing the huge ethical and moral dangers threatening this nation. In the late 1950's, when hospitals were first starting to experience these serious financial losses, it forced hospital administrators to develop Regional Planning and Cost Containment Programs — and in 1979, this author, as a hospital administrator and the Chair Person of a Regional Cost Containment Committee, spent a full day with Gerald Ford, a former President of the United States, seeking his advice on how we might return to a single non-profit prepayment healthcare system. Senator Gerald Ford and Governor George Romney and I had become friends when I first moved my HSI research to Lansing, Michigan — where the two of them and myself, a hospital Administrator of the first to be "Class One Emergency Center" at the St. Lawrence Hospital, implemented the "State's Disaster Program" during Michigan's record breaking snow storm of 1976. After my meeting with former President Gerald Ford ended, he put his arm over my shoulder and said:

John, the health care system will have to collapse before things will get better.

I didn't believe him then, but I do now, as our healthcare costs are skyrocketing out of control. However, one thing I'm now noticing is that both Congress and our Presidential candidates are starting to discuss returning to a single cost effective healthcare system. And for the first time in the history of the United States, one of our Senators, the Honorable Bernie Sanders, has recently attempted to openly expose these many serious problems that are destroying this nation's Democracy.

Today's many decentralized profit seeking insurance programs and the decentralized computer development in healthcare are only digging a deeper hole with their disorganized variety of computers, software, and computer operating systems that will only make it far more difficult when we are eventually forced to return to a comprehensive single cost effective database solution to today's healthcare dilemma. The following description of a single comprehensive computer network will hopefully help Americans to understand the enormous job that lies ahead.

INTRODUCTION

Health Systems Institute, a non-profit organization, had long ago coordinated the research and design of a single health record database communications network Master Plan — involving the voluntary work of over one thousand physicians, nurses and paraprofessionals from the Universities of Michigan State, Minnesota, Iowa, Michigan, Kentucky, and British Columbia. HSI also surveyed some 250 private hospitals and clinics in trying to determine what was needed to design a comprehensive single computer health record network that could improve today's healthcare system. A government study, by "The Department of Health, Education and Welfare" reported: *"This research and educational orientation of the [HSI] project suggests that the impact of this system will be far reaching"* — however, many of this nation's politicians have ignored this HSI research that attempted to develop a Master Plan for healthcare because of the donations they receive from this powerful profit seeking insurance business and the pharmaceutical industry. They do not seem to realize that a professional human service requires cooperation ... not competition; standards ... rather than deregulation; and centralization ... not decentralization

NATIONAL DATABASE NETWORK STANDARDS

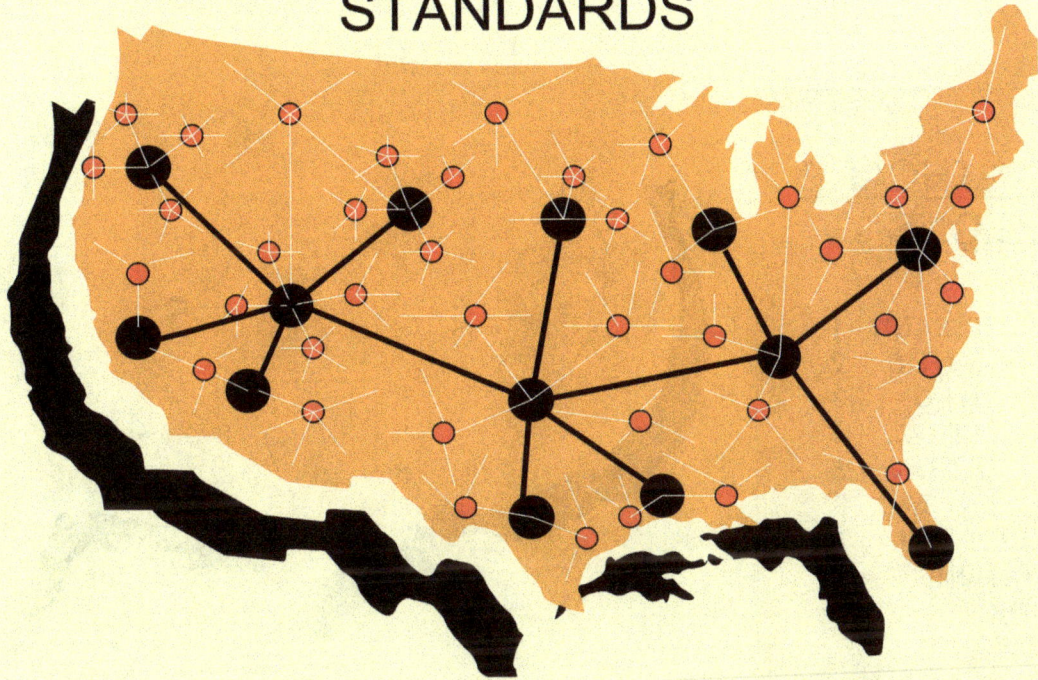

National Standards

In a communications network, confidential patient information must remain the legal property of the patient, and yet be instantly available at the patient's request … to any accredited healthcare facility, clinic, or licensed physician's office throughout the United States. It appears that a few Congressmen are finally seeing the cost effectiveness of such a network, but we do need to be sure they fully understand the cost and size of the master plan required to accomplish this vitally important service for our sick and indigent. They also need to recognize that substantial federal and philanthropic support will be required to meet the hardware, software and operating system's communications network requirements. One thing for sure, this country can no longer delay this decision much longer and we cannot expect our financially drained sick and disabled to pay for such a major development.

REGIONAL STANDARDS

HEALTHCARE REGIONS

NEW ENGLAND	1
MID ATLANTIC	2
S. ATLANTIC	3
E.S. CENTRAL	4
E.N. CENTRAL	5
W.N. CENTRAL	6
W.S.CENTRAL	7
MOUNTAIN	8
PACIFIC	9

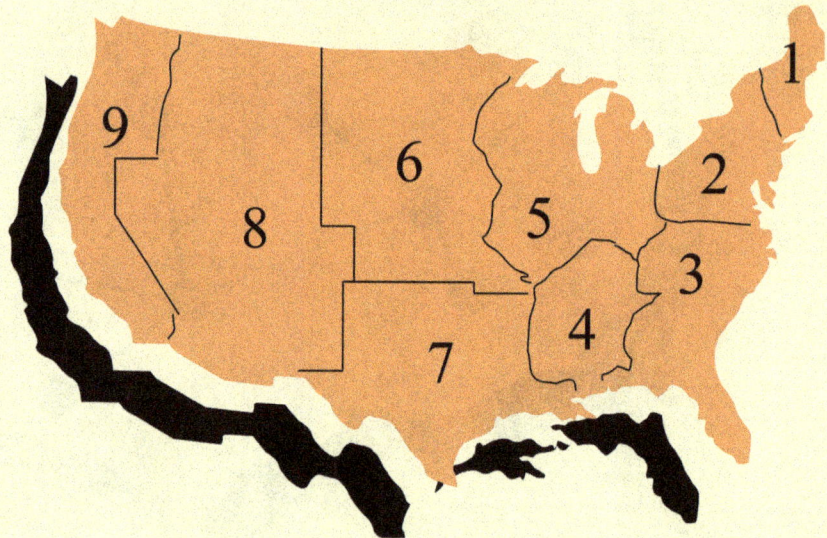

Regional Standards

A compatible community, region, and nationwide communications network requires the AHA, the AMA, the Joint Commission on Accreditation of Health Care Organizations, all specialty organizations, and all participating healthcare facilities in all nine healthcare regions, to cooperate in the development of such standards.

REGIONAL COMMUNICATION STANDARDS

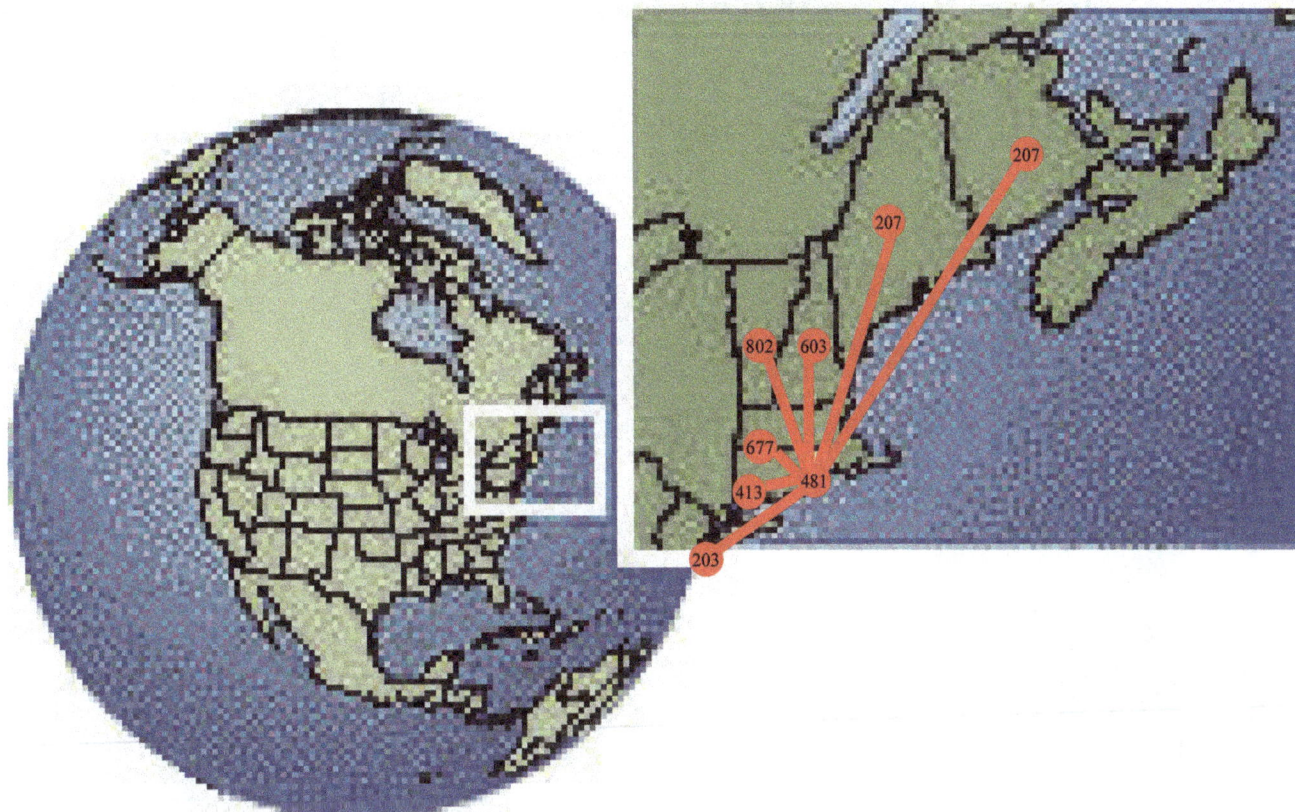

Regional Facility Standards

Health record applications should first be designed and tested in one selected region. For example: A legally confidential patient master population file is essential in eliminating the costly duplication of patient registration at every facility. To accomplish this, proper identification of the patient is the first step in creating a health record database, and it requires a standard communication network that can provide full redundancy at the local, regional, and national level.

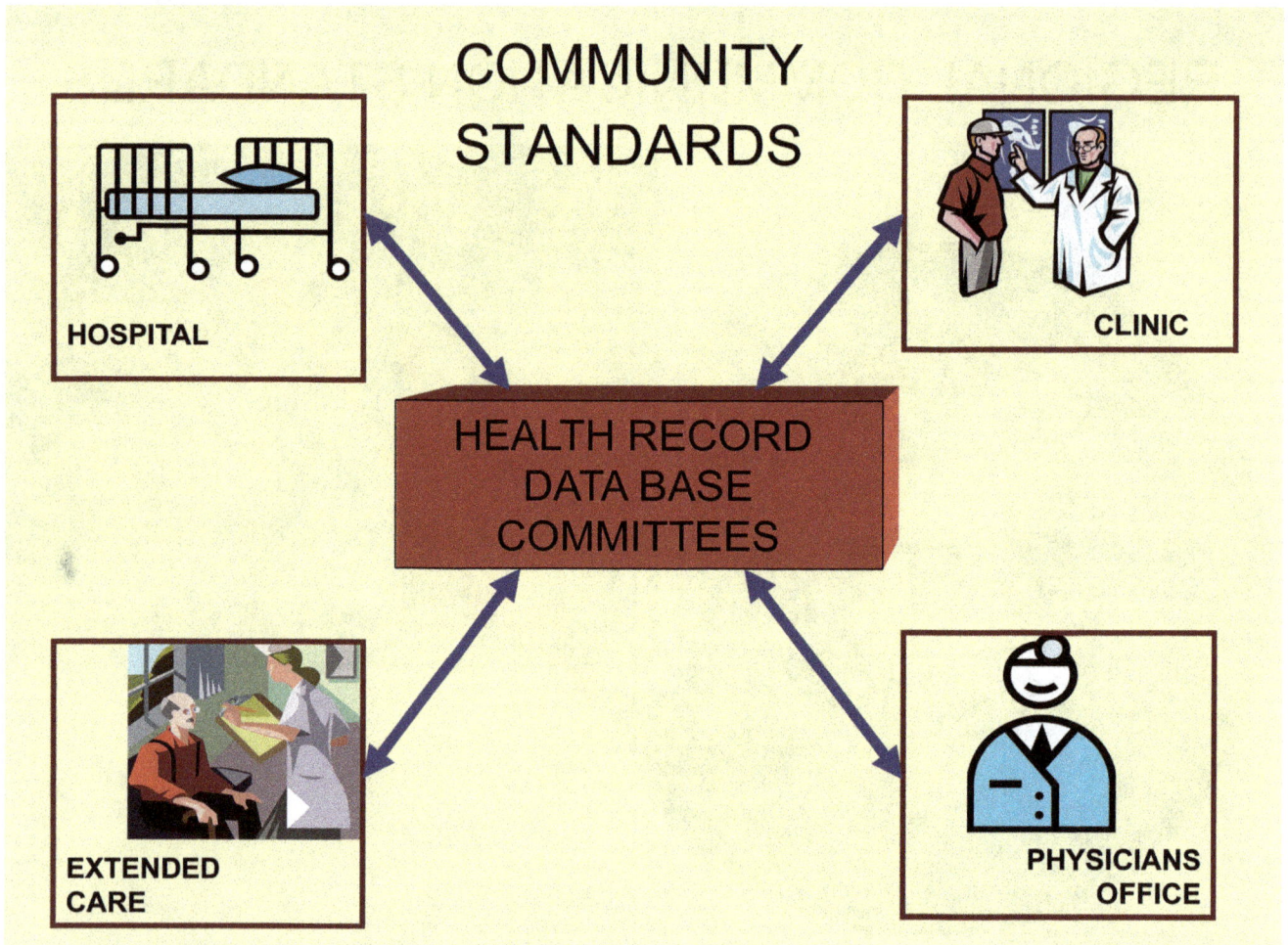

COMMUNITY STANDARDS

HOSPITAL

CLINIC

HEALTH RECORD
DATA BASE
COMMITTEES

EXTENDED
CARE

PHYSICIANS
OFFICE

Community Standards

Physician's committees need to coordinate their work within the community, such as the hospitals, clinics, physician's offices, and the extended care facilities.

PHYSICIAN HEALTH RECORD STANDARDS   NURSING HEALTH RECORD STANDARDS

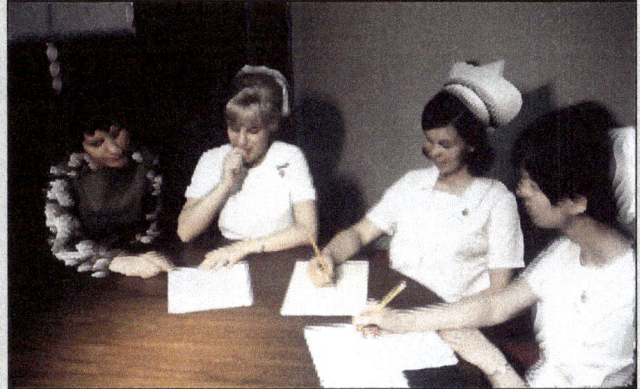

Physicians and Nursing Health Record Standards

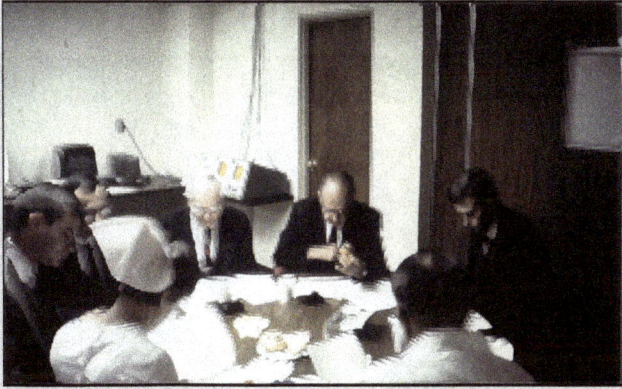

Here you see one of the original physician committees that volunteered their time to define the complex order and observation files and library standards, so they could someday rely on a paperless medical record. A nurse and a programmer then transferred the doctor's decisions to a touch CRT terminal, where they could test their decisions on something other than paper. The CRT terminal you see in the background was the first touch sensitive terminal ever built in the United States, for which HSI wrote the specs, and Control Data Corporation built what they called the "Digiscribe". Bill Norris, President of Control Data, volunteered to build the Digiscribe at no cost to HSI. With the Digiscribe, each medical specialty then had to define their specific orders and observations, their physical exam; their problem, symptom and diagnostic categories; their updates and progress notes; and all the related libraries and files standards for each medical record application. HSI used a technically trained nurse to coordinate and confirm the physician's decisions. Nursing committees were also required to design their observations; progress notes; comparative flow charts; and their update application standards as well as their libraries and files. They also confirmed their decisions on the CRT, prior to replacing the paper documents.

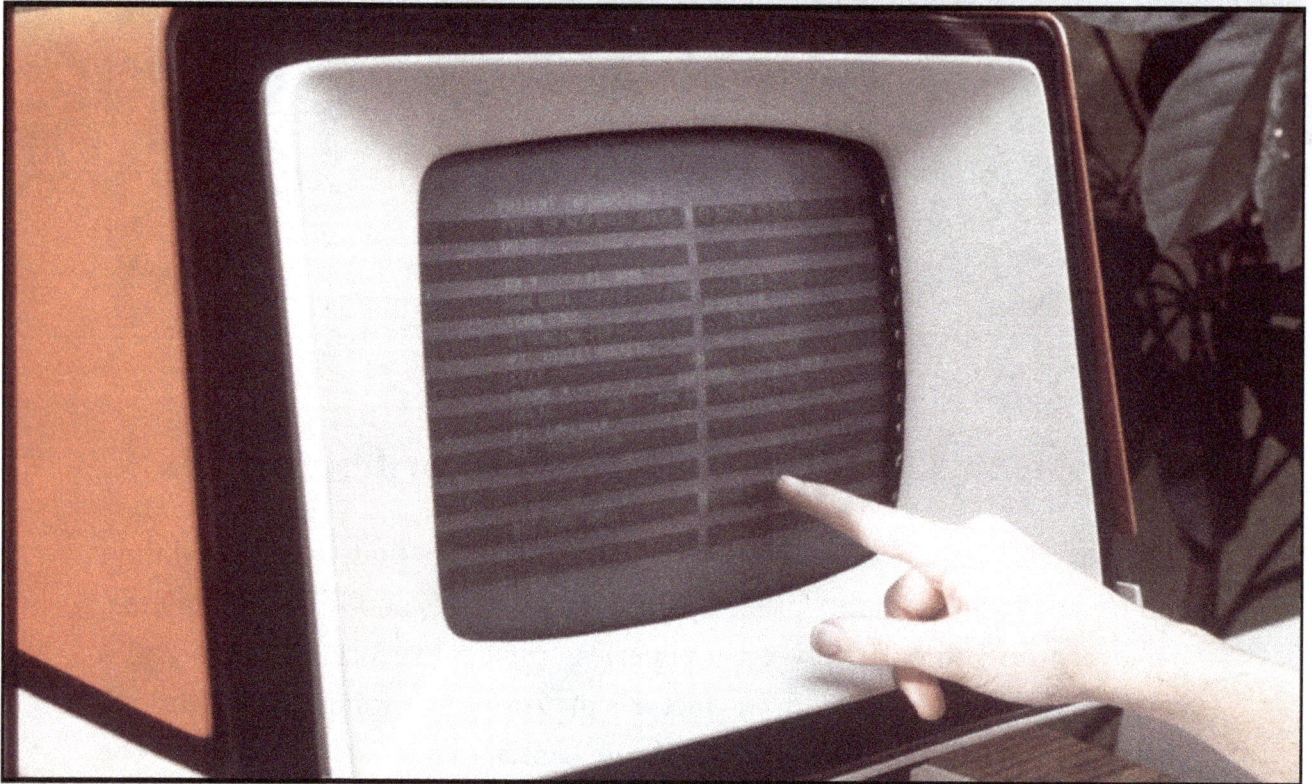

Touch Terminal Standards

Physicians and nurses did not like to type. This is why HSI asked Control Data to develop a human interface that required they just point at the screen. Doctor Ian Brown, a neurologist said: ***Doctors can be very intelligent in some respects, but they can be rather stupid in others. They're much like infants ... they just like to point at what they want.*** As a result, CDC invented the first touch sensitive terminal, which proved very acceptable to both the nurses and doctors. Later, the mouse proved acceptable, but the touch terminal lent itself more readily to structured entry, which reduced errors and allowed retrospective database and statistical analysis ... important in clinical audit. Since clinical orders and diagnostic libraries and files could be structured, the Digiscribe was the preferred interface. HSI later developed a code generator that used structured entry to generate the actual application programs by computer, cutting application software development costs by an estimated 90 percent.

THE KEYBOARD STANDARDS

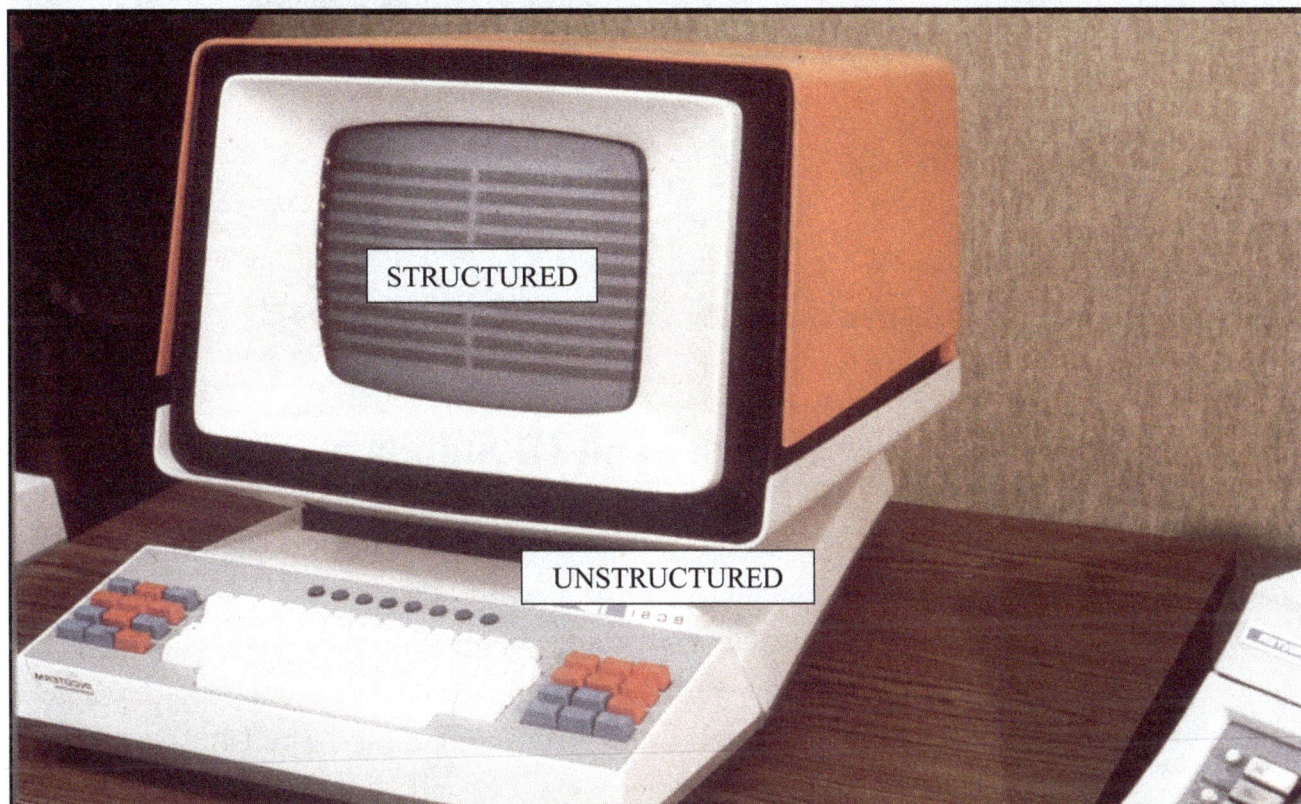

STRUCTURED

UNSTRUCTURED

The Keyboard Standards

The keyboard allowed for unstructured entry, and had a special library key that was used to obtain educational material within selected application circuits. For example: If the doctor was ordering a drug, they could review the drug detailing, the incompatibilities of drug to drug, or drug to lab, or even review a text without going to the library. The same held true if they were ordering an x-ray or a lab, they could always obtain a standard educational description. The user could also page forward or backward on the CRT, simply by touching that key. If the user was qualified, he or she could obtain a hard copy of a display by simply touching the print key.

PRINT STANDARDS

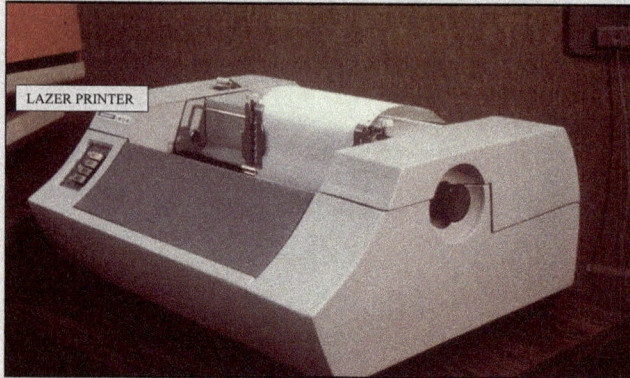

LAZER PRINTER

ID STANDARDS

CARD READER

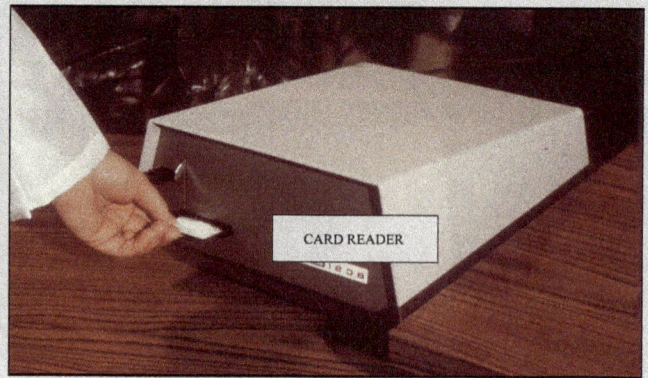

The Laser Printer and ID Standards

A Laser printer was essential on the nursing station, where noise was unacceptable and paper documents were usually discouraged whenever possible. Remote, hand carried and fixed bedside input devices will eventually totally replace paper worksheets for the nurse and doctor of the future, eliminating note pads, pencils, and errors of memory. The Unit Dose cart for administering patient medications cut all types of monthly medication errors from over 300 to an average of 3 per month.

Initially a card reader was used to identify each user, but this was later changed to a "Think Lock" that asked each user a series of changing personal questions, before gaining access to the system. In the future, eye, palm, or fingerprint may prove preferable.

USER STANDARDS-MASTER FILE

PERSONNEL APPLICATIONS AND CIRCUITS	ADMITTING SUPERVISOR	ADMITTING CLERK	PHYSICIAN A	NURSE	TYPIST
REGISTRATION	●	●			
ENTER REGISTRATION	●	●			
CONFIRM ARRIVAL	●	●			
REVISE REGISTRATION	●	●			
SCHEDULING	●	●			
REVISE SCHEDULE	●	●			
BED ASSIGNMENT	●	●			
UPDATE WAITING LIST	●	●			
ACCESS MEDICAL RECORD			●	●	●
READ HISTORY			●	●	
ENTER HISTORY			●	●	●
ENTER PHYSICAL			●	●	
PROBLEM LIST			●	●	●
ETC.					

User Standards-Master

All healthcare personnel should be trained and assigned applications and sub-circuits under a position control application called, "The User Master File," which must be maintained under strict management control by each facility. Patient confidentiality should be restricted by circuit assignment, which allows only authorized positions to utilize assigned circuits.

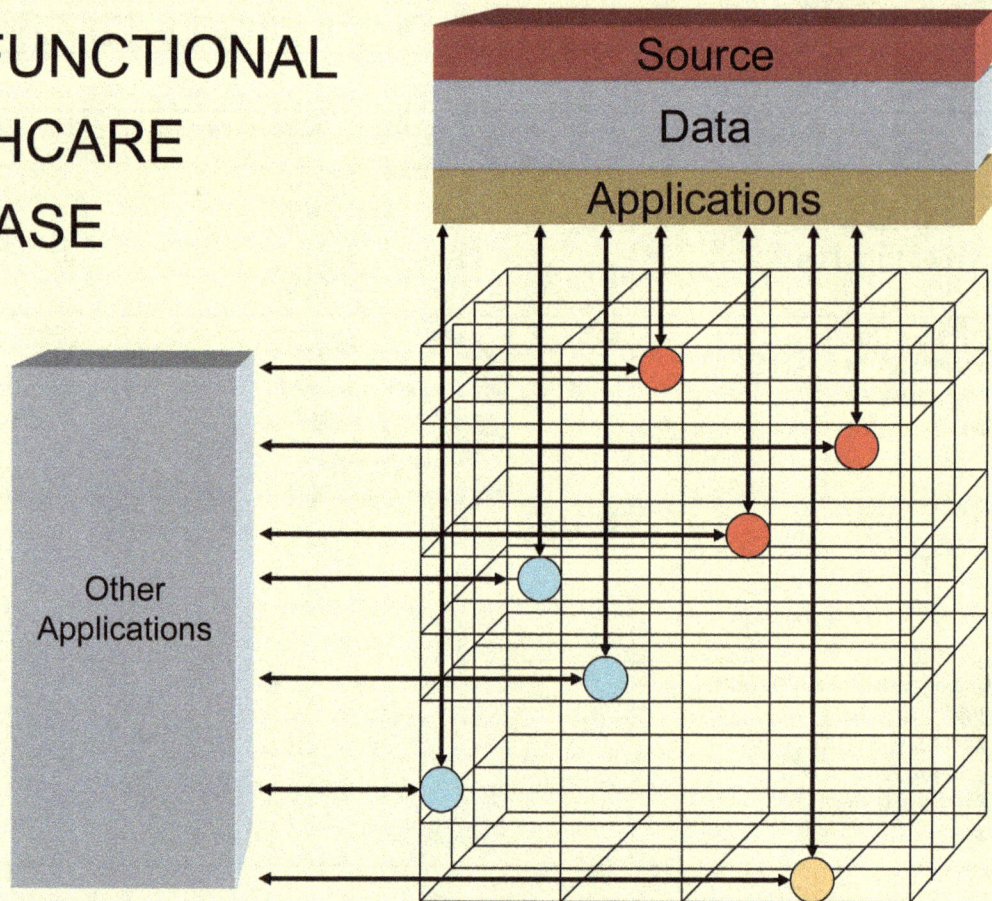

Multifunctional Healthcare Database

Capturing patient information where it first occurs eliminates errors and the costly repeating of patient information over and over. Capturing all patient information at source point can be accomplished when the patient first registers, when a health professional confirms a patient observation for a diagnosis, treatment, examination or procedure, or when a licensed physician places an order.

PATIENT SOURCE DATA INCLUDES

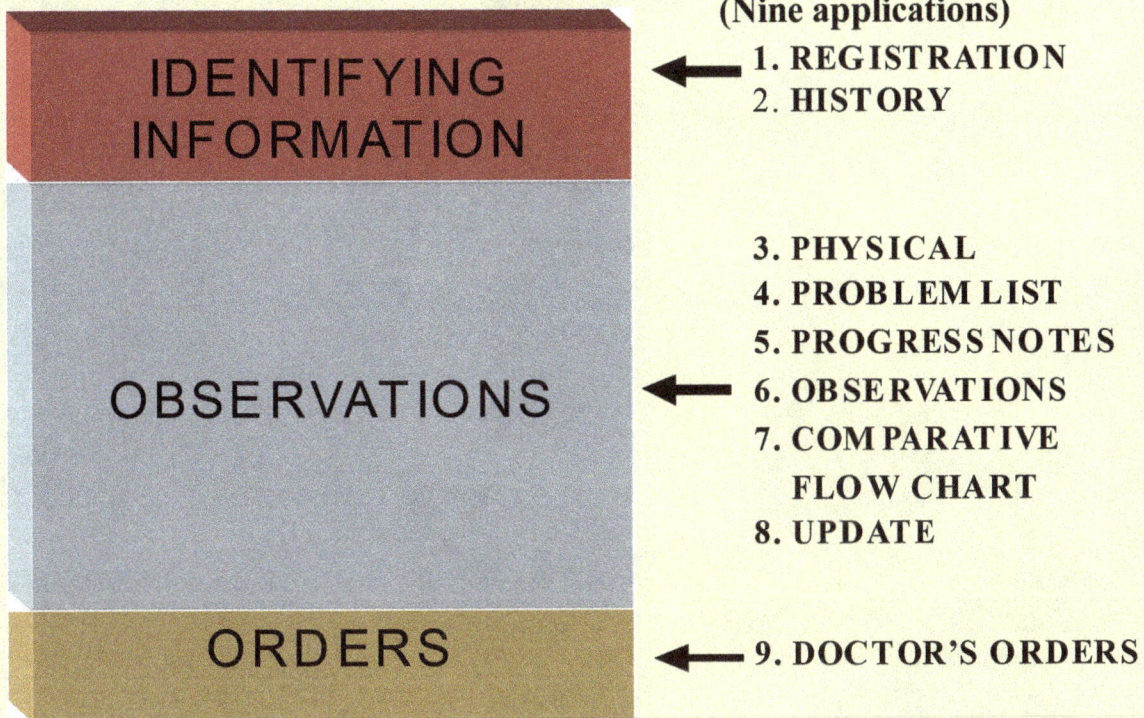

(Nine applications)

IDENTIFYING INFORMATION	← 1. REGISTRATION 2. HISTORY
OBSERVATIONS	3. PHYSICAL 4. PROBLEM LIST 5. PROGRESS NOTES ← 6. OBSERVATIONS 7. COMPARATIVE FLOW CHART 8. UPDATE
ORDERS	← 9. DOCTOR'S ORDERS

Patient Source Data-ID-Observations-Orders

Capturing patient information where it first occurs at its source eliminates errors and the costly repeating of patient information over and over. Capturing all patient information at source point can be accomplished when the patient first registers, when a health professional confirms a patient observation for a diagnosis, treatment, examination or procedure, or when a licensed physician places an order. The patient's medical record is made up of nine applications. The patient's Registration and History applications provide all patient identifying information. The Observations made by a nurse or physician includes six additional source data applications: The Physical Examination; the Problem/Diagnostic list; the doctor and nurse's Observations and Progress Notes, and their Update Reports; and the Comparative Analog Flow Charts. A doctor or a registered nurse can enter the Physician's Orders, however all orders entered by an RN require physician confirmation within a prescribed period of time, and this may be accomplished from any terminal within the network

REGISTRATION STANDARDS

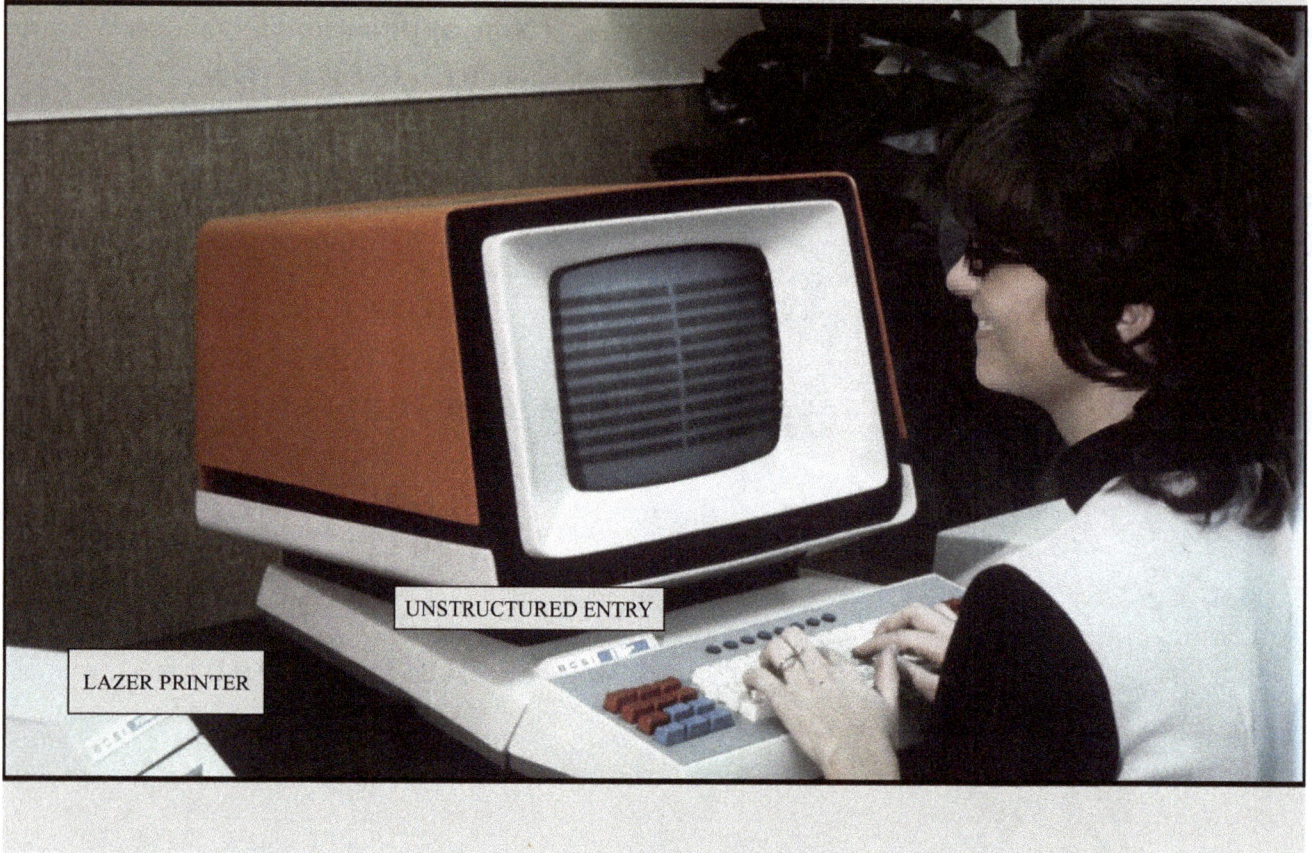

LAZER PRINTER

UNSTRUCTURED ENTRY

Typed Registration Standards

The registration clerk types all unstructured ID information into a "Master Population File" at the time of the patient's initial treatment or admission. Upon entering unstructured information, a typist will interview each non-emergent patient prior to admission, treatment, or examination, confirming all typed entry information as correct and current.

PATIENT REGISTRATION STANDARD

UNSTRUCTURED REGISTRATION ENTRY FORMAT

Pt. Name:_____(30)_____ Pt. #:_____(12)_____ Pt. Rm & Bed #:__(5)__ Clinical Flag Codes:____(6)____

Address:_____(50)_____ Attending Phy._____(14)____ Cons. Phy:___(14)___

Date:___(8)____ Time:___(4)___ Birth Date:____(8)____ Race:_(1)_ Religion:__(4)__ Sex:_(1)_ Marital Status:__(1)__

Social Security #:_____(11)_____

Patient's Employer:_____(50)_____

Responsible Party:_____(30)_____ Relation:_(4)_ S.S. # :_____(11)_____

Legal Responsible Party:____(Pt, R.P- if other, add name & add.)_____

Emergency Contact:_____(LRP, FRP, Other)_____ Relation:__(4)____

Financial Responsible Party:__(PT, LRP, or FRP)_____

FRP Address:_____(50)_____ Phone #:_____(12)_____

Employer:_____(38)_____

Prepayment Program:_____ Prepayment #_____

PP Address:_____(50)_____ Phone #:_____(12)_____

Registration Form

After the initial registration, the registration clerk will only update the patient's Master Population File. HSI used structured entry for religion, race, sex, marital status, prepayment parties, and physicians, while date and time were automatically assigned. Before each episode of treatment, the Clerk will update the patient's registration information prior to the patient receiving additional treatment, examination or orders.

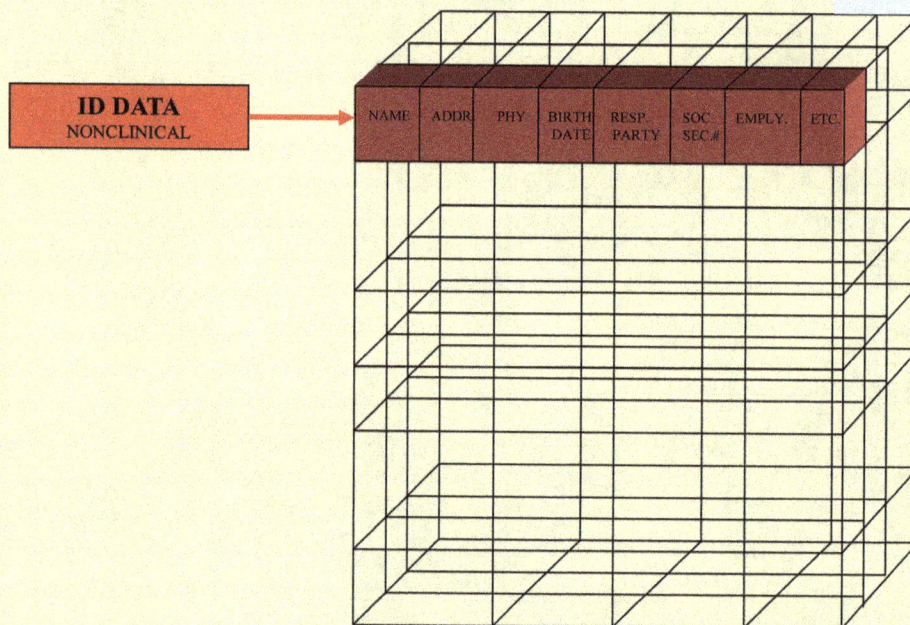

Enter ID into Database

At the patient's first registration all ID information is entered into the patients database Master Population File by date, database, to be used by all health care facilities treating or examining the patient.

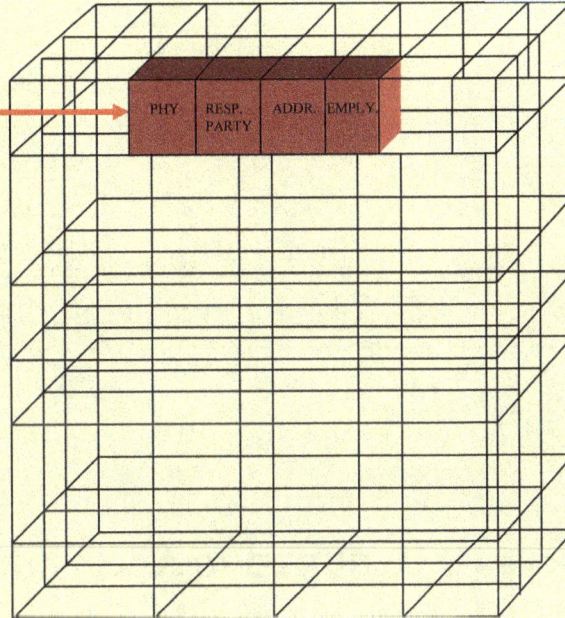

Revising ID Database

Thereafter, the registration clerk can revise ID information by date after reviewing the database and confirming any revisions. Here the user revises physician, the responsible party, address, and employer by date.

ACCESS HEALTH RECORD STANDARDS

User Identification

Select Access Health Record

Select Patient Name

Select Patient Name
👉 <u>204-1 Smith, Sally Q.</u>
242-1 Jones, Timothy, F.

Users ID Required to Access the Medical Record

All health record applications require a physician, nurse or paraprofessional be properly identified in the User File before gaining access through an attending physician's order in the patient's medical record. Physicians are also assigned appropriate medical record circuits by staff privileges … as maintained in the Medical Staff Index Standards. Upon selecting "Access a Health Record" the physician or health professional can only gain access to those registered patients they previously ordered admission, treatment, examination or consultation for. In an emergency, where there is no ID information, a patient record can be started with a John Doe ID, and registration will then be completed at a later time but here again an admission order by the attending physician is required. Then a list of patients the user is actively treating will be shown. Here, a physician selects Sally Q Smith.

ACCESS
HEALTH
RECORD
STANDARDS

User Identification

Select Access Health Record

Select Patient Name

204-1 Smith, Sally Q.

242-1 Jones, Timothy, F.

Enter History	Review History
Enter Physical	Review Physical
Enter Problem List	Review Problem List
Enter Progress Notes	Review Progress Notes
Enter Nurse Observations	Review Comp. Flow Chart
Enter Orders	Review Dr. Nurse Updates

Select Enter or Review a Medical Record Application

A physician would then be able to enter or review all active application circuits for Sally Q. Smith's medical record.

ACCESS
HEALTH
RECORD
STANDARDS

User Identification

Select Access Health Record

Select Patient Name

204-1 Smith, Sally Q.

242-1 Jones, Timothy, F.

Enter History   Review History

Patient History

A patient, for example, would only be allowed to enter or review a history.
In this case, the patient, or their designate, selects enter history.

Patient Name: 204-1 Smith, Sally Q.

SELECT ONE METHOD TO ENTER HISTORY

DICTATION INSTRUCTIONS

TYPED ENTRY

STRUCTURED QUESTIONNAIRE

Active	■ Exit	☐ Forward	☐ Print
Keys	☐ Entry	☐ Reverse	☐ Library

Structured Questionnaire

A patient could "Enter or Review" their History and in this case the patient, or their designate, selects to enter their history using the Structured Questionnaire. If a paraprofessional or nurse were entering the History for a patient, they could also choose to dictate or type an unstructured history. The average time to complete the initial history using a touch terminal is approximately 20 minutes.

```
Patient Name:   204-1 Smith, Sally Q.


SELECT ONE HISTORY CATEGORIE:


CHIEF COMPLAINT

PREVIOUS MEDICAL HISTORY

FAMILY HISTORY

SOCIAL HISTORY


                              Touch Exit Key When Complete
```

| Active | ■ Exit | ☐ Forward | ☐ Print |
| Keys | ☐ Entry | ☐ Reverse | ☐ Library |

Chief Complaint

The user would then select a History Category such as Chief Complaint, Previous Medical History, Family History, or Social History. The previous history identifies hospitalizations, operations, disease indexes, deaths and general family history, while the social history obtains marital status, employment, habits and other general information. Here the user selects Chief Complaint.

```
  I AM NOW HAVING TROUBLE WITH:        Select One or Continue

  PAIN                            MY EARS

  DIZZY SPELLS OR  BLACKOUTS      MY NOSE, MOUTH OR THROAT

  HEADACHES                       MY STOMACH & SWALLOWING

  MY EMOTIONS            👉        MY LUNGS AND BREATHING

  MY NERVES                       ALLERGY

  SPEECH OE COORDINATION          CIRCULATION OF BLOOD

  MY EYES                         MY INTESTINES AND BOWELS

                                  CONTINUE
```

Active	▮ Exit	▯ Forward	▯ Print
Keys	⊔ Entry	▮ Reverse	▯ Library

My Lungs and Breathing

Next, the patient would be asked what their problem is. Here they select, My Lungs and Breathing. Had they touched continue, they could review additional problem categories.

```
MY LUNGS & BREATHING
_____

 WHAT IS THE PROBLEM?

 Select One


 COUGHING                        INFECTION OR PNEUMONIA

 SHORT OF BREATH                 SMOKING

 SPITTING UP BLOOD               SPITTING UP PHLEGM

 WHEEZING                        NONE OF THESE
```

Active	■ Exit	☐ Forward	☐ Print
Keys	☐ Entry	■ Reverse	☐ Library

Short of Breath

You will note that each selection accumulates at the top of the display, and in this case the user selects Short of Breath.

<u>MY LUNGS & BREATHING SHORT OF BREATH WHILE CLIMBING STAIRS OR AWAKENED FROM SLEEP</u>

WHEN ARE YOU SHORT OF BREATH?

<u>Select One or Multiple</u>

CLIMBING STAIRS

DOING LIGHT WORK

AWAKEND FROM SLEEP

AT REST OR SITTING STILL

CONTINUE

Active	■ Exit	☐ Forward	☐ Print
Keys	☐ Entry	■ Reverse	☐ Library

Climbing Stairs-Awakened from Sleep

Note the change in selecting one or multiple. Here the user selects while "Climbing Stairs" and "Awakened From Sleep" and then the user selects continue. The patient actually records his or her selections with the computer adding the appropriate prefix and suffix where necessary.

LOGIC SEQUENCE

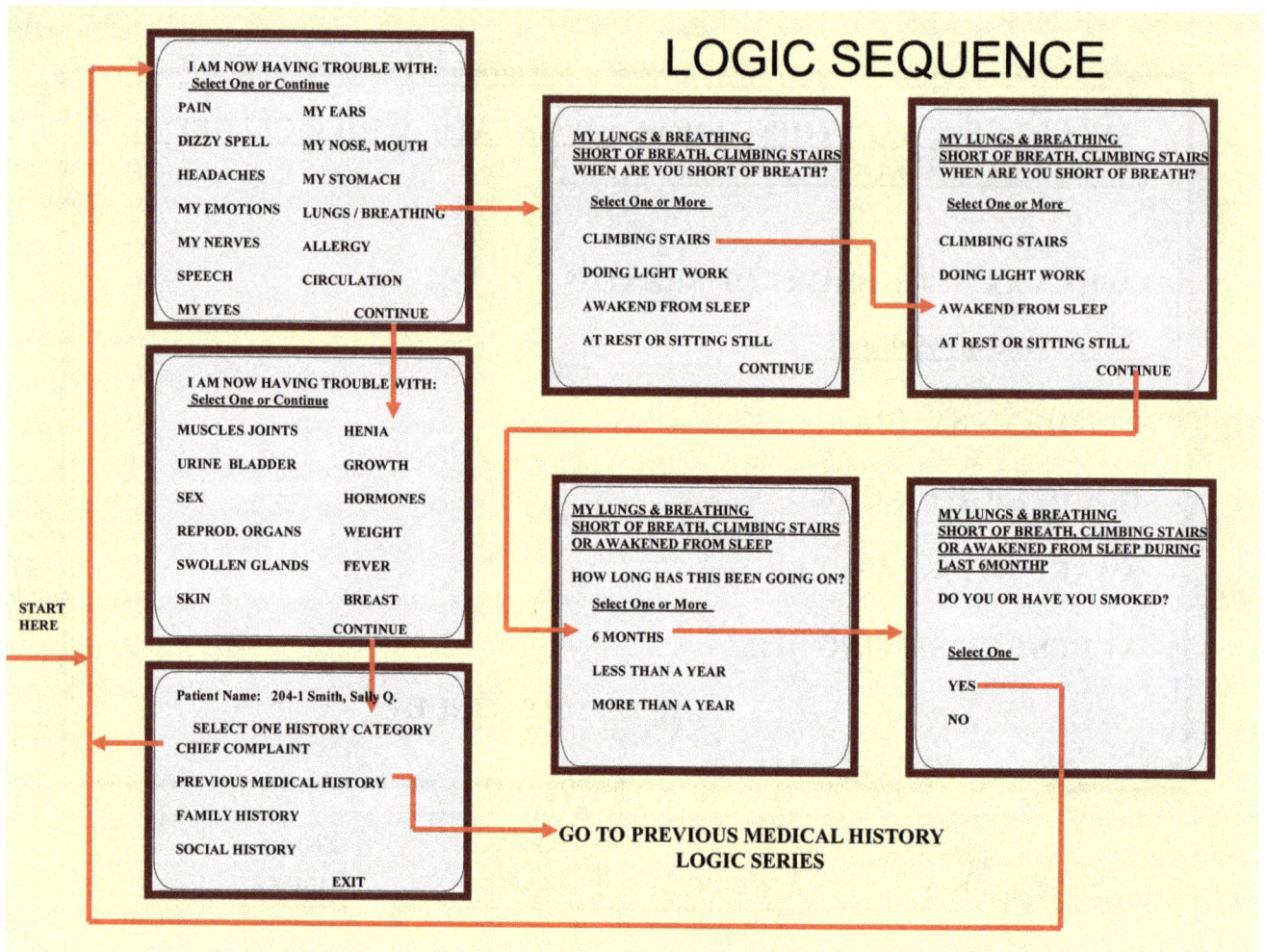

I AM NOW HAVING TROUBLE WITH:
Select One or Continue

PAIN	MY EARS
DIZZY SPELL	MY NOSE, MOUTH
HEADACHES	MY STOMACH
MY EMOTIONS	LUNGS / BREATHING
MY NERVES	ALLERGY
SPEECH	CIRCULATION
MY EYES	CONTINUE

MY LUNGS & BREATHING
SHORT OF BREATH, CLIMBING STAIRS
WHEN ARE YOU SHORT OF BREATH?

Select One or More

CLIMBING STAIRS

DOING LIGHT WORK

AWAKEND FROM SLEEP

AT REST OR SITTING STILL

CONTINUE

MY LUNGS & BREATHING
SHORT OF BREATH, CLIMBING STAIRS
WHEN ARE YOU SHORT OF BREATH?

Select One or More

CLIMBING STAIRS

DOING LIGHT WORK

AWAKEND FROM SLEEP

AT REST OR SITTING STILL

CONTINUE

I AM NOW HAVING TROUBLE WITH:
Select One or Continue

MUSCLES JOINTS	HENIA
URINE BLADDER	GROWTH
SEX	HORMONES
REPROD. ORGANS	WEIGHT
SWOLLEN GLANDS	FEVER
SKIN	BREAST
	CONTINUE

MY LUNGS & BREATHING
SHORT OF BREATH, CLIMBING STAIRS
OR AWAKENED FROM SLEEP

HOW LONG HAS THIS BEEN GOING ON?

Select One or More

6 MONTHS

LESS THAN A YEAR

MORE THAN A YEAR

MY LUNGS & BREATHING
SHORT OF BREATH, CLIMBING STAIRS
OR AWAKENED FROM SLEEP DURING
LAST 6MONTHP

DO YOU OR HAVE YOU SMOKED?

Select One

YES

NO

Patient Name: 204-1 Smith, Sally Q.

SELECT ONE HISTORY CATEGORY
CHIEF COMPLAINT

PREVIOUS MEDICAL HISTORY

FAMILY HISTORY

SOCIAL HISTORY

EXIT

START HERE

GO TO PREVIOUS MEDICAL HISTORY
LOGIC SERIES

Series of History Displays

By selecting My Lungs and Breathing, the user has been guided through a series of logic displays relating to that problem. Physicians can tailor these displays to their specialty for each problem they treat. Once the patient completes the Chief Complaint series, they would then complete their Previous Medical History, Family History, and Social History by following similar sequential displays that accumulate into a complete message. (See the HSI History Manual) Remember the patient actually records his or her selections with the computer adding the appropriate prefix and suffix where necessary.

MY LUNGS & BREATHING ARE SHORT OF BREATH WHEN
CLIMBING STAIRS OR AWAKENED FROM SLEEP OVER
THE LAST SIX MONTHS, AND I HAVE PREVIOUSLY SMOKED

CONFIRMED   NOT CONFIRMED

| Active | ▉ Exit | ☐ Forward | ▉ Print |
| Keys | ☐ Entry | ▉ Reverse | ☐ Library |

My Lungs and Breathing Summary

All selections accumulate into a complete statement for confirmation by
date. Here you see the accumulative message for My Lungs and Breathing.
If a previous history exists, the patient will only be asked to make changes
or additions. When the user confirms the statement, they then will go on to
complete the entire history, which will then be filed in the patient's
database. You will note the patient can also use the print key to obtain a hard
copy if desired.

MULTIFUNCTIONAL HEALTHCARE DATABASE

History Database

In this example, the patient has revised their family history, social history, and they have a new chief complaint, which is stored in the database by date.

ACCESS HEALTH RECORD STANDARDS

| User Identification |
| Select Access Health Record |

Select Patient Name

204-1 Smith, Sally Q.

242-1 Jones, Timothy, F.

Enter History	Review History
Enter Physical	Review Physical
Enter Problem List	Review Problem List
Enter Progress Notes	Review Progress Notes
Enter Nurse Observations	Review Comp. Flow Chart
Enter Orders	Review Dr. Nurse Updates

Enter Physical

Once the physician is identified they select Access Health Record and then select the patient from a list of their patients as shown here. Here a physician or their designate can enter a physical exam by selecting, Enter Physical.

```
Patient Name:  204-1 Smith, Sally Q.              SELECT ONE

VITAL SIGNS                          NECK
GENERAL APPEARANCE                   LYMPH NODES
SKIN                                 CHEST AND LUNGS
HEAD                                 HEART
EXTERNAL EYE                         BREAST
INTERNAL EYE                         ABDOMEN
EARS                                 BACK
NOSE AND NASOPHARYNX                 PELVIC
OROPHARYNX                           CRANIO SACRAL
RECTAL                               NEOUROLOGY
PELVIC                               EXTREMETIES
MALE GENITALIA                       GENERAL




                                     SELECTIONS COMPLETE
```

Active	▌ Exit	☐ Forward	☐ Print
Keys	☐ Entry	☐ Reverse	☐ Library

General Appearance

A physician can complete the physical exam on a touch terminal, or a paraprofessional may enter the findings from the physician's notes for later confirmation by the attending physician in the Update application, within a designated time period. Here the physician selects, General Appearance.

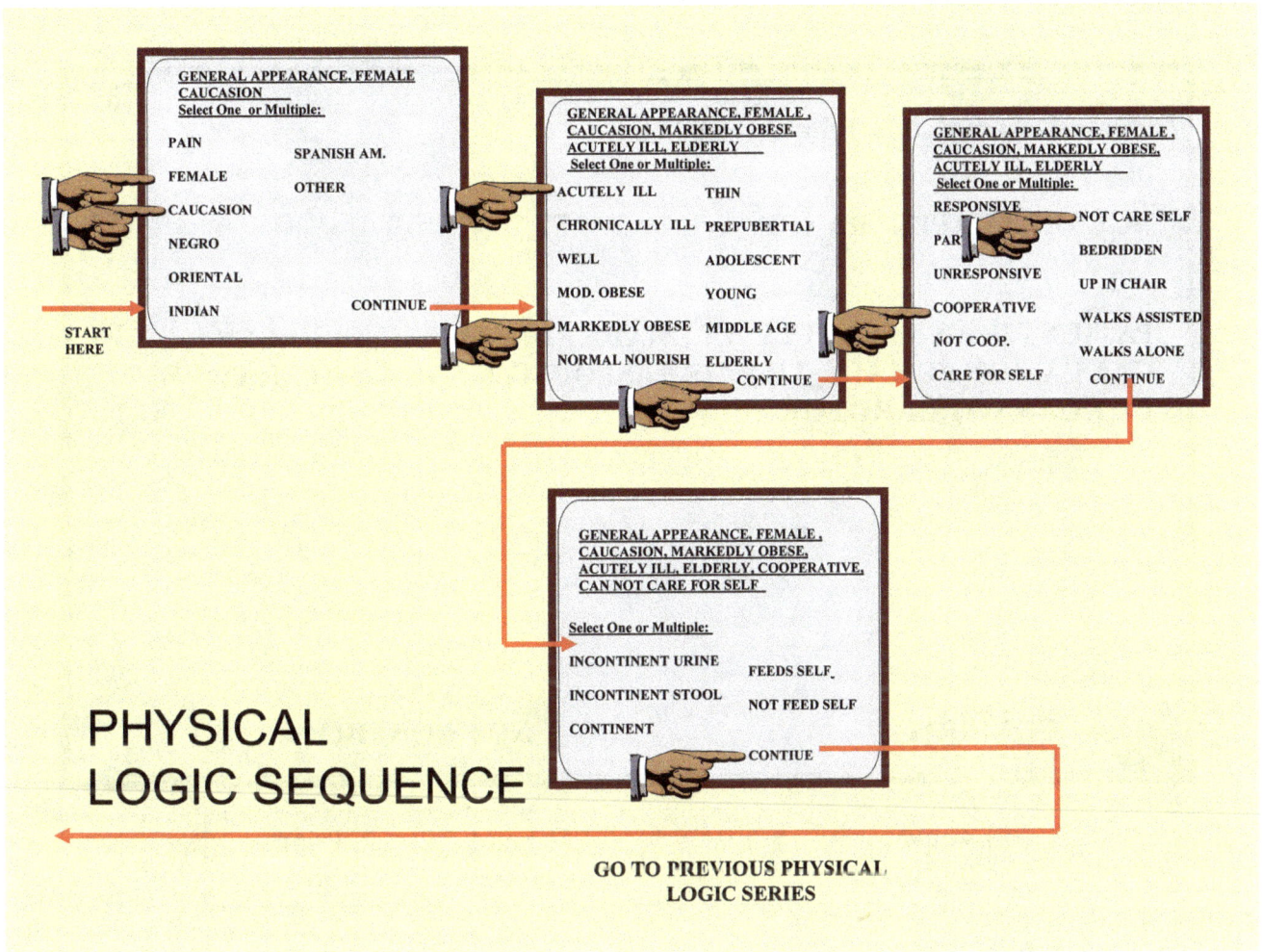

GENERAL APPEARANCE, FEMALE
CAUCASION
Select One or Multiple:

PAIN   SPANISH AM.

FEMALE   OTHER

CAUCASION

NEGRO

ORIENTAL

INDIAN   CONTINUE

START
HERE

GENERAL APPEARANCE, FEMALE,
CAUCASION, MARKEDLY OBESE,
ACUTELY ILL, ELDERLY
Select One or Multiple:

ACUTELY ILL   THIN

CHRONICALLY ILL   PREPUBERTIAL

WELL   ADOLESCENT

MOD. OBESE   YOUNG

MARKEDLY OBESE   MIDDLE AGE

NORMAL NOURISH   ELDERLY
                   CONTINUE

GENERAL APPEARANCE, FEMALE,
CAUCASION, MARKEDLY OBESE,
ACUTELY ILL, ELDERLY
Select One or Multiple:

RESPONSIVE   NOT CARE SELF

PAR   BEDRIDDEN

UNRESPONSIVE   UP IN CHAIR

COOPERATIVE   WALKS ASSISTED

NOT COOP.   WALKS ALONE

CARE FOR SELF   CONTINUE

GENERAL APPEARANCE, FEMALE,
CAUCASION, MARKEDLY OBESE,
ACUTELY ILL, ELDERLY, COOPERATIVE,
CAN NOT CARE FOR SELF

Select One or Multiple:

INCONTINENT URINE   FEEDS SELF

INCONTINENT STOOL   NOT FEED SELF

CONTINENT

                       CONTIUE

PHYSICAL
LOGIC SEQUENCE

GO TO PREVIOUS PHYSICAL
LOGIC SERIES

Physical Logic Series

Once again the physician completes a series of sequential questions relating to the patient's General Appearance. The Physician can also tailor these displays to their specialty for each body system examined, with the computer adding appropriate prefix and suffix in the accumulated message.

Patient Name: 204-1 Smith, Sally Q.

GENERAL APPEARANCE:

PATIENT IS AN ACCUTELY ILL, MARKEDLY OBESE, ELDERLY CAUCASION FEMALE, THAT IS RESPONSIVE AND COOPERATIVE BUT CANNOT CARE FOR SELF.

CONFIRM   **NOT CONFIRM**

Active	■ Exit	☐ Forward	☐ Print
Keys	☐ Entry	☐ Reverse	☐ Library

General Appearance

After completing the General Appearance questions, the accumulative structured entry is confirmed as accurate and the physician is returned to the next category to select another body system … or to exit.

MULTIFUNCTIONAL HEALTHCARE DATABASE

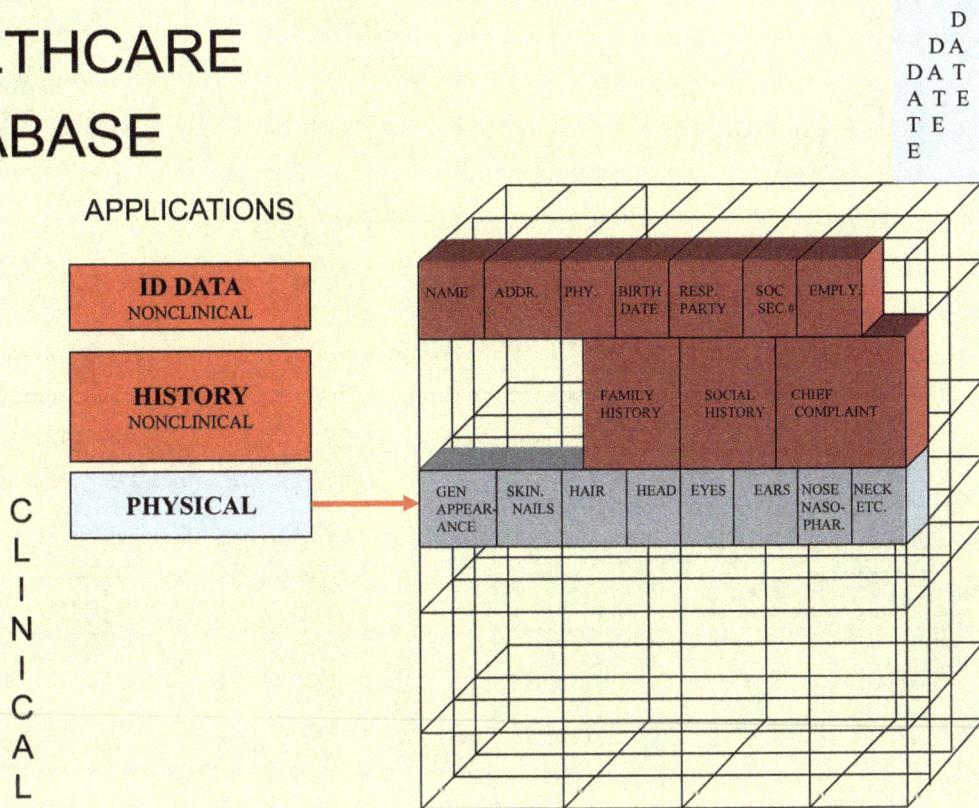

APPLICATIONS

ID DATA
NONCLINICAL

HISTORY
NONCLINICAL

| PHYSICAL |

C L I N I C A L

D D A DA T DA A T E T E E

| NAME | ADDR. | PHY. | BIRTH DATE | RESP. PARTY | SOC SEC.# | EMPLY. |

| FAMILY HISTORY | SOCIAL HISTORY | CHIEF COMPLAINT |

| GEN APPEAR-ANCE | SKIN. NAILS | HAIR | HEAD | EYES | EARS | NOSE NASO-PHAR. | NECK ETC. |

Physical Exam Entry to Database

When the attending or consulting physician completes the physical exam, those data elements are added to the database on the date it was completed, however, if a nurse or designate completed the exam, the licensed attending physician is required to confirm the physical exam in the attending physician's update application before entry into the database by date.

ACCESS HEALTH RECORD STANDARDS

User Identification

Select Access Health Record

Select Patient Name

204-1 Smith, Sally Q.

242-1 Jones, Timothy, F.

Enter History	Review History
Enter Physical	Review Physical
Enter Problem List	Review Problem List
Enter Observations, Flow Chart, or Progress Notes	Review Progress Notes
	Review Comp. Flow Chart
Enter Orders	Review Dr. Nurse Updates

Enter a Problem/Diagnosis

A physician or his designate can also enter a problem, symptom, or diagnosis by selecting, "Enter a Problem".

SELECT ONE:

PHYSICIAN'S QUICK LIST

TYPE IN A PROBLEM

CATEGORICAL LIST OF PROBLEMS

Active	■ Exit	☐ Forward	☐ Print
Keys	☐ Entry	■ Reverse	☐ Library

Selecting Problem Category

Here the user selects the Categorical List of Problems. HSI used the current HICDA International Code of Disease reference library for its Categorical List, however some specialists may prefer to create their own specialty problem or diagnosis quick list.

```
SELECT ONE:

INFECTIOUS DISEASE              UROGENITAL

NEOPLASMS                       SKIN SUBCUTIS

ENDO. METAB./BLOOD DISEASE      MUSCULOSKELETAL

NERVIOUS SYSTEM                 CONGENITAL NEONATAL DIS.

EYE, EAR                        SIGNS & SYMPTOMS

CARDIOVASCULAR                  INJURIES

RESPIRATORY                     ADVERSE EFFECTS

DIGESTIVE
```

| Active | ■ Exit | ☐ Forward | ☐ Print |
| Keys | ☐ Entry | ■ Reverse | ☐ Library |

Selects Cardiovascular Category

Here the user selects Cardiovascular.

SELECT ONE:

CARDIOVASCULAR HEART FAILURE

ATRIAL FIBRILLATION

PROXIMAL TACHYCARDIA

LEFT VENTRICAL FAILURE

VENTRICULAR FIBRILATION

CARDIAC ARREST

OTHER DISEASES OF RHYTHM

HEART BLOCK

| Active Keys | ■ Exit | ☐ Forward | ☐ Print |
| | ☐ Entry | ■ Reverse | ☐ Library |

Selects Heart Failure

Then the user selects Cardiovascular Heart Failure.

__05/05__

TYPE IN MONTH AND YEAR ONLY

Active	■ Exit	▢ Forward	▢ Print
Keys	▢ Entry	■ Reverse	▢ Library

Date of Onset

The user then elects to type May 5th as the date of onset, and then presses the entry key. HSI also used a month and year selection table, which was preferred over typed entry.

SMITH, SALLY # 01-712-056-907

 # 01   CARDIOVASCULAR HEART FAILURE- Code 270.0

ONSET	ENTRY	STATUS
05/05	05/20	ACTIVE

CONFIRM   NOT CONFIRM

Active	■ Exit	□ Forward	□ Print
Keys	□ Entry	■ Reverse	□ Library

Confirms Problem

The user then "Confirms" the patient's number one active problem of Cardiovascular Heart Failure, which is automatically coded as #270.0, with the date of onset stated to be May 5th, as entered on May 20th. Remember, a diagnosis is a clinical decision that only a licensed physician can make.

MULTIFUNCTIONAL HEALTHCARE DATABASE

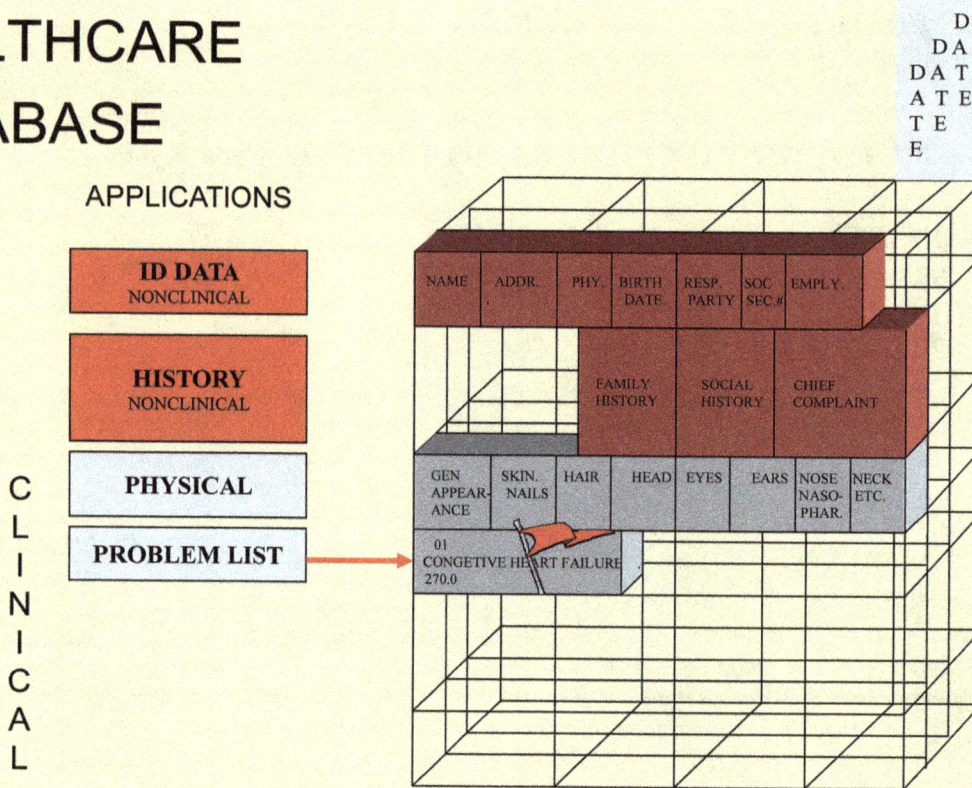

Enters Problem/Diagnosis into Database

Problem 01, Congestive Heart Failure is then entered into the database, with the computer automatically assigning the active diagnosis code as #270.0. If entered by an authorized registered nurse, the physician update will flag the doctor to confirm the nurse's entry in his update application within a predefined time limit, as shown here. Remember, the physician may use any terminal at any location, even their office terminal to confirm a nurse's entry. Errors are frequently made in today's manual system, when a patient is treated without a diagnosis or a problem statement. Timely entry and convenient confirmation of a diagnosis will go a long way in reducing errors.

User Identification

Select Access Health Record

Select Patient Name

204-1 Smith, Sally Q.

242-1 Jones, Timothy, F.

Enter History	Review History
Enter Physical	Review Physical
Enter Problem List	Review Problem List
Enter Observations, Flow Chart, or Progress Notes	Review Progress Notes
	Review Comp. Flow Chart
Enter Orders	Review Dr. Nurse Updates

Observations

Entering a doctor or nurse observation or a progress note, or creating a patient flow chart, comprises a major part of the observation database. The HSI committees found that almost all types of observations could be entered through structured entry, involving specially designed libraries and files that were developed by the health professionals themselves. The advantage of structured entry was that all data could later be statistically analyzed accurately, which will someday have an enormous advantage to the current inept and cost prohibited manual entry and analysis we currently live with. Physician's found that almost all radiological reports, operative reports, and even progress notes could be pre-structured with only minimal variations sometimes being typed in.

SELECT ONE:

    ENTER VITAL SIGNS

    ENTER PHYSICAL OBS.

    ENTER EMOTIONAL OBS.

    ENTER ABNORMAL OBS.

    TYPE IN OBSERVATION

    ENTER PROGRESS NOTES

Active Keys	■ Exit ☐ Entry	☐ Forward ■ Reverse	☐ Print ☐ Library

Progress Notes

Here the physician decides to enter their progress notes. Almost every specialty will customized the observation progress notes to some level of structured entry, once they became familiar with the system.

```
Patient Name:   204-1 Smith, Sally Q.


SELECT ONE METHOD TO ENTER PROGRESS NOTES



DICTATION INSTRUCTIONS

TYPED ENTRY

STRUCTURED ENTRY
```

Active	■ Exit	□ Forward	□ Print
Keys	□ Entry	□ Reverse	□ Library

Dictation Entry

The physician or their designate could also type or dictate if they choose to do so. The overall goal however is to eliminate unstructured hand written observations or orders that are often illegible and can cause serious misinterpretations or errors. Here a physician elects to enter a progress note after making daily rounds. Vital signs entries were almost always structured and later reviewed on an analog or bar graph report, whereas physical, emotional, and abnormal observations were often typed or dictated instead of being structured.

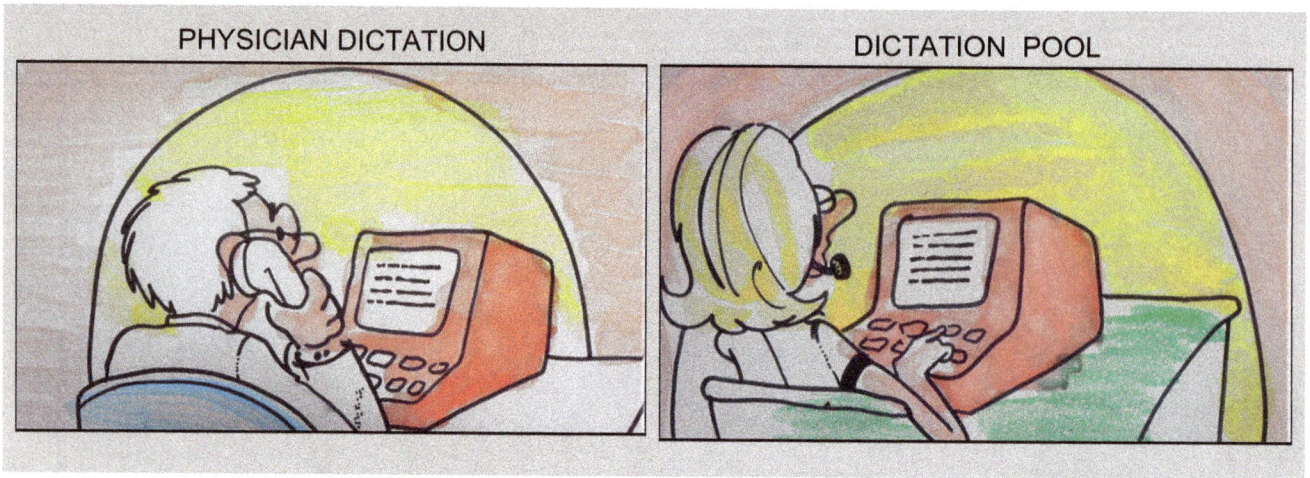

PHYSICIAN DICTATION   DICTATION POOL

Physician's Dictation – Pool Typing

An on line head set at each terminal is used to communicate the physician's dictated message to a central dictation pool where they are required to enter the message into the system within a specified time standard, where it will be later confirmed in the physician's update application before final entry into the patient's database.

STRUCTURED PROGRESS NOTES

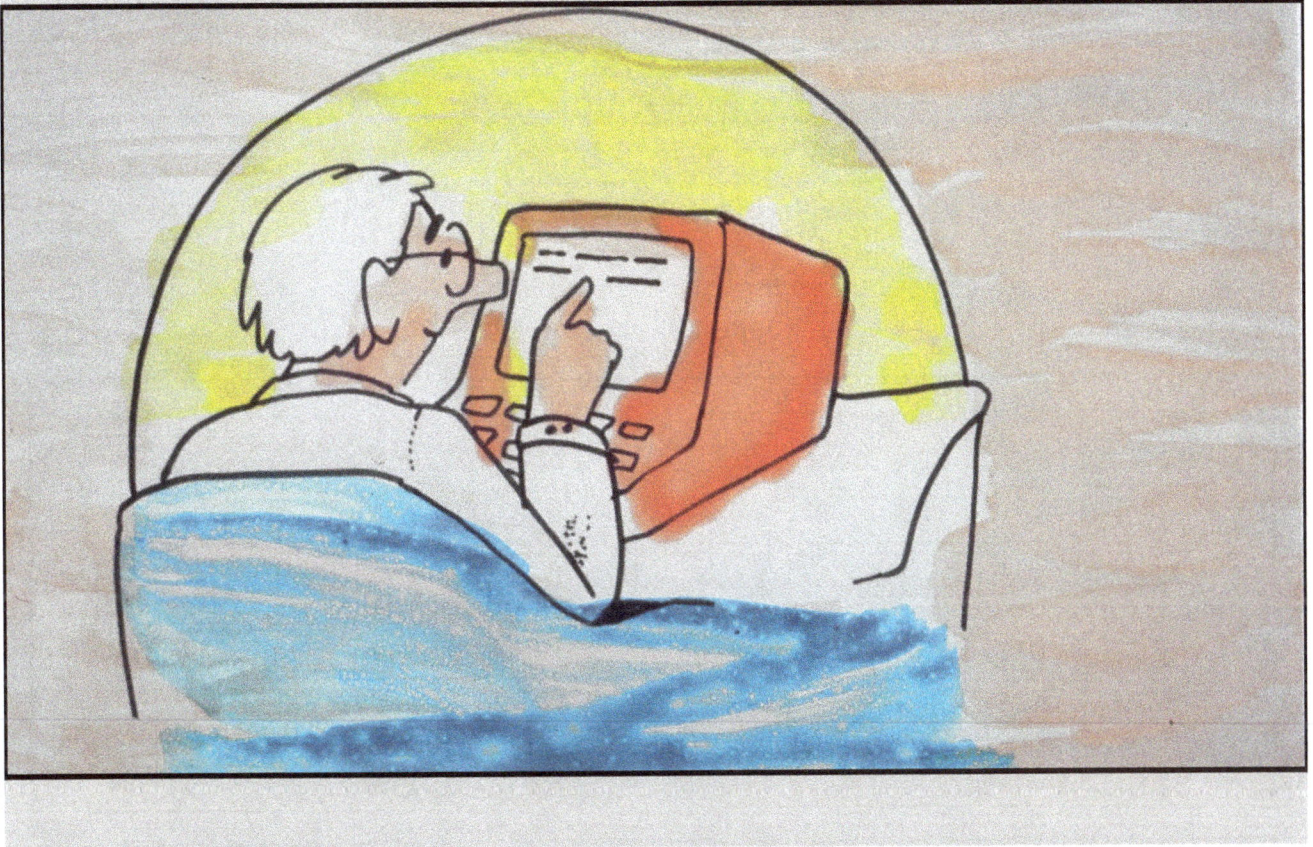

Structured Progress Notes

Physicians wanting to use structured entry will need to customize their own routine progress notes. Specialty reports form X-ray and Lab and Ancillary Services, operative reports, and routine progress notes can readily be structured, with dictation used as needed. Physicians can also readily inter-mix dictation with structured entry whenever necessary.

ACCESS HEALTH RECORD STANDARDS

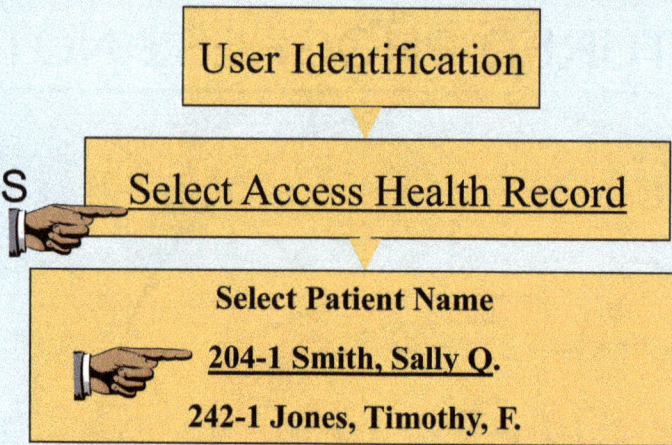

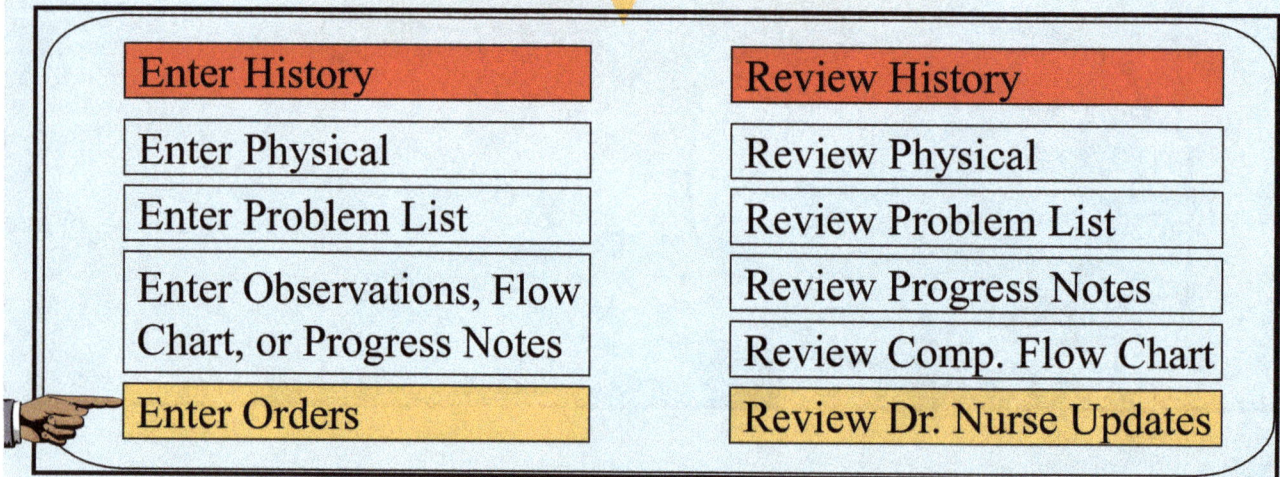

| User Identification |

| Select Access Health Record |

Select Patient Name

204-1 Smith, Sally Q.

242-1 Jones, Timothy, F.

Enter History	Review History
Enter Physical	Review Physical
Enter Problem List	Review Problem List
Enter Observations, Flow Chart, or Progress Notes	Review Progress Notes
	Review Comp. Flow Chart
Enter Orders	Review Dr. Nurse Updates

Enter an Order

Entering orders is a very important application, and the physician should be the one to enter their order whenever possible. A phone order, to a registered nurse, requires the physician to confirm each order in their update application within a predefined time standard. Remember, if the physician's office is on line, they can easily enter or confirm orders from that location.

```
   SELECT ONE:


ORDER QUICK LIST

TYPE IN AN ORDER

ORDER LIBRARY
```

Active	■ Exit	☐ Forward	☐ Print
Keys	☐ Entry	■ Reverse	☐ Library

Order Library

Here a physician selects the Order Library or they could call up their own Order Quick List, or they can type in an order as desired.

```
SELECT ONE CATEGORIE:


        LABORATORY                ANESTHESIA

👉     PHARMACY                   OCCUPATIONAL THERAPY

        NURSE'S INSTRUCTIONS       PHYSICAL THERAPY

        RADIOLOGY                 SOCIAL SERVICE

        CARDIOPULMONARY           CONSULTATION

        SURGERY                   TRANSFER SERVICE
```

Active	■ Exit	☐ Forward	☐ Print
Keys	☐ Entry	■ Reverse	☐ Library

Pharmacy Order

Here the user selects the Pharmacy Order. You will note they have numerous choices where the user could also select a consulting physician, nursing, ancillary departments, surgery or even transfer the patient.

SELECT ONE DRUG CATEGORY:

CENTRAL NERVOUS SYSTEM

CARDIOVASCULAR

AUTONOMIC

ANTINEOPLASTIC

ANTI-INFECTIVE AGENT

ANTIHISTAMINE

ELECTROLITIC/CALORIC/AND WATER BALANCE

Active	■ Exit	☐ Forward	☐ Print
Keys	☐ Entry	■ Reverse	☐ Library

Order by Drug Category

Under the formulary the physician select the Electrolytic/Caloric, and Water Balance drug category.

```
SELECT ONE:


ORDER BY FORMULARY

ORDER BY ALPHABETIC FORMULARY

ORDER PERENTERAL FLUIDS
```

Active	■ Exit	☐ Forward	☐ Print
Keys	☐ Entry	■ Reverse	☐ Library

Order by Formulary

Here the physician or his designate selects to order by Formulary. If someone other than the physician orders for the doctor, the attending physician will need to approve the order in his update application before the order can be accomplished.

```
SELECT ONE SUBCATEGORY:

  ACIDIFYING AGENTS

  REPLACEMENT SOLUTIONS

  CALORIC AGENTS

  SALT AND SUGAR SUBSTITUTES

  DIURETICS
```

Active	■ Exit	☐ Forward	☐ Print
Keys	☐ Entry	■ Reverse	☐ Library

Diuretics

The physician next selects Diuretics.

```
  SELECT ONE:


  BENURON   (BENDROFLUMETHAZIDE)

  EXNA  (BENZTHIAZIDE)

  NEOHYDRIN  (CHLORM EDODRIN)

  DIURIL (CHLORATHIAZIDE)

  HYGROTON  (CHLORTHALIDONE)

  ANHYDRON  (CYCLOTHIAZIDE)

  EDECRIN  (ETHACRYNIC ACID)
```

Active Keys	■ Exit	☐ Forward	☐ Print
	☐ Entry	■ Reverse	☐ Library

Edecrin

The Physician then selects Edecrin.

```
  EDUCATIONAL DISPLAY FOR EDECRIN

SELECT ONE:


COMMODITY PROFILE          ☞ DOSE AND ADMINISTRATION

USE AND EFFICACY             PHARMACEUTICS

DRUG COMBINATIONS            METOBOLISM

MECHANISM OF ACTION          TOXICOLOGY

WARNINGS
```

Active Keys	■ Exit □ Entry	□ Forward ■ Reverse	□ Print ■ Library

Dose & Administration & Library Key

Note: The drug library key is active on this display, and the user touches dose and administration and then the library key and receives an educational display on the recommended dose and administration of Edecrin.

```
EDECRIN (ETHACRYNIC ACID)
 DOSE AND ADMINISTRATION

Adults- 1st day; 50 to 100 mg given as a single dose after a meal; 12 to 24
hours should be allowed to assess the effect of the initial dose.

Second day; If no response to the initial dose, the daily dose should be
increased to 100mg given in two doses.

Third day; 100 mg can be administered in the morning, and 50 to 100 mg
May be administered after noon or evening meal, depending on the response
to the morning dose.

Further adjustments may be made on 25-50 mg increments.
Total daily dose should not exceed 400 mg.

                              👉  CONTINUE
```

Active Keys	■ Exit ■ Entry	☐ Forward ■ Reverse	☐ Print ■ Library

Library Education Display

The advantage of having this type of information immediately available will have a significant impact on improving the quality of drug administration and drug errors and reactions will be reduced significantly. Too many busy physicians ignore this step today, because it's just not convenient, and this is where errors can occur.

SELECT EDECRIN DRUG FORM:

TABLET ORAL

SUSPENSION ORAL

INJECTIBLE-IM

INJECTABLE-IV

| Active | ■ Exit | ☐ Forward | ☐ Print |
| Keys | ☐ Entry | ■ Reverse | ■ Library |

Tablet Oral

After reviewing the drug detailing, the physician selects tablet oral.

```
EDECRIN (ETHACRYNIC ACID)
TABLET ORAL
50 MG.                          225 MG.

75 MG.                          250 MG.

100 MG.                         275 MG.

125 MG.                         300 MG.

150 MG.                         325 MG.

175 MG.                         350 MG.

200 MG.                         375 MG.

                                OTHER
```

Active Keys	■ Exit □ Entry	□ Forward ■ Reverse	□ Print ■ Library

Dosage 50 MG

At this point, each selection now accumulates at the top of the display, and the physician then selects the 50-milligram dosage.

```
EDECRIN (ETHACRYNIC ACID)
TABLET ORAL-50 MG.-
_____


FREQUENCY

INITIAL DOSE FOLLOWED BY:

ONCE DAILY

DAILY PC

BID PC
                                          OTHER
```

Active	▪ Exit	▫ Forward	▫ Print
Keys	▫ Entry	▪ Reverse	▪ Library

Frequency

Here they select the frequency, as BID PC.

```
EDECRIN (ETHACRYNIC ACID)
TABLET ORAL-50 MG.-BID PC- 3 DAYS


SELECT  DURATION:

24 HOURS                                    5 DAYS

1 DAY                                       6 DAYS

2 DAYS                                      7 DAYS

3 DAYS

4 DAYS
```

Active Keys	■ Exit ☐ Entry	☐ Forward ■ Reverse	☐ Print ■ Library

Duration

The user selects for the duration of 3 days.

MULTIFUNCTIONAL HEALTHCARE DATABASE

APPLICATIONS

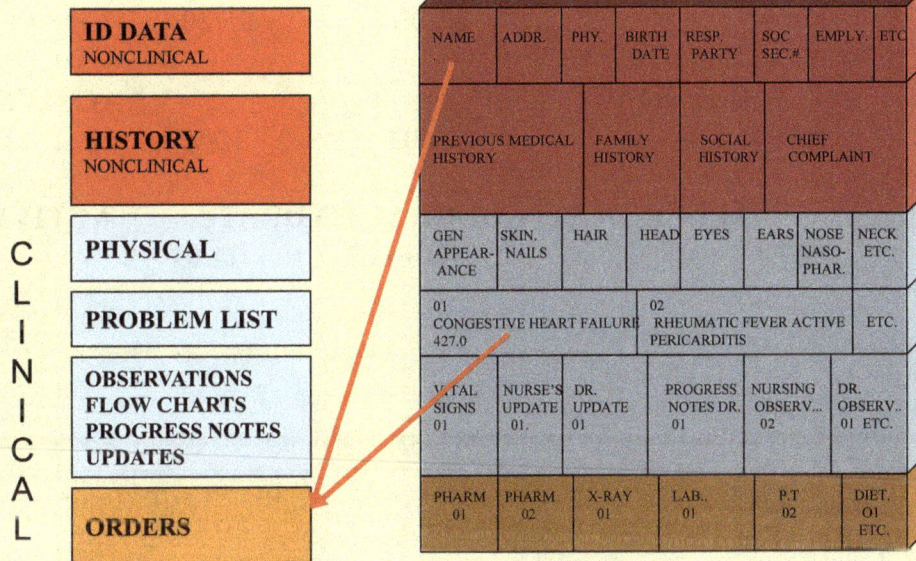

| ID DATA
NONCLINICAL |
| HISTORY
NONCLINICAL |
| PHYSICAL |
| PROBLEM LIST |
| OBSERVATIONS
FLOW CHARTS
PROGRESS NOTES
UPDATES |
| ORDERS |

C L I N I C A L

D DA DA TE A T E E

| NAME | ADDR. | PHY. | BIRTH DATE | RESP. PARTY | SOC SEC.# | EMPLY. | ETC |

| PREVIOUS MEDICAL HISTORY | FAMILY HISTORY | SOCIAL HISTORY | CHIEF COMPLAINT |

| GEN APPEAR-ANCE | SKIN, NAILS | HAIR | HEAD | EYES | EARS | NOSE NASO-PHAR. | NECK ETC. |

| 01 CONGESTIVE HEART FAILURE 427.0 | 02 RHEUMATIC FEVER ACTIVE PERICARDITIS | ETC. |

| VITAL SIGNS 01 | NURSE'S UPDATE 01. | DR. UPDATE 01 | PROGRESS NOTES DR. 01 | NURSING OBSERV... 02 | DR. OBSERV. 01 ETC. |

| PHARM 01 | PHARM 02 | X-RAY 01 | LAB.. 01 | P.T 02 | DIET. 01 ETC. |

Checks Database

Upon completing the drug order, the database will automatically show the patient's ID and Problem list … so the user can select which patient problem is being treated.

```
SMITH, SALLY   01-712-056-907
SELECT PROBLEM FOR EDECRIN ORDER:

PROB. #              NAME                          STATUS
       CODE                  ONSET        ENTRY

# 01          CARDIOVASCULAR HEART FAILURE    ACTIVE
       270.0                 05/05          05/20

#02             OBESITY                         ACTIVE
       277.0                 10/03          10/03

#03          ALLERGICTO CHLORAL HYDRATE       ACTIVE
       967.1                 11/01          11/01
```

Active	∎ Exit	☐ Forward	☐ Print
Keys	☐ Entry	∎ Reverse	☐ Library

Problem One

Here the physician selects problem one for the Edecrin order, which is Cardiovascular Heart Failure, code 270.0. Note: this display shows the entire patient's problem list.

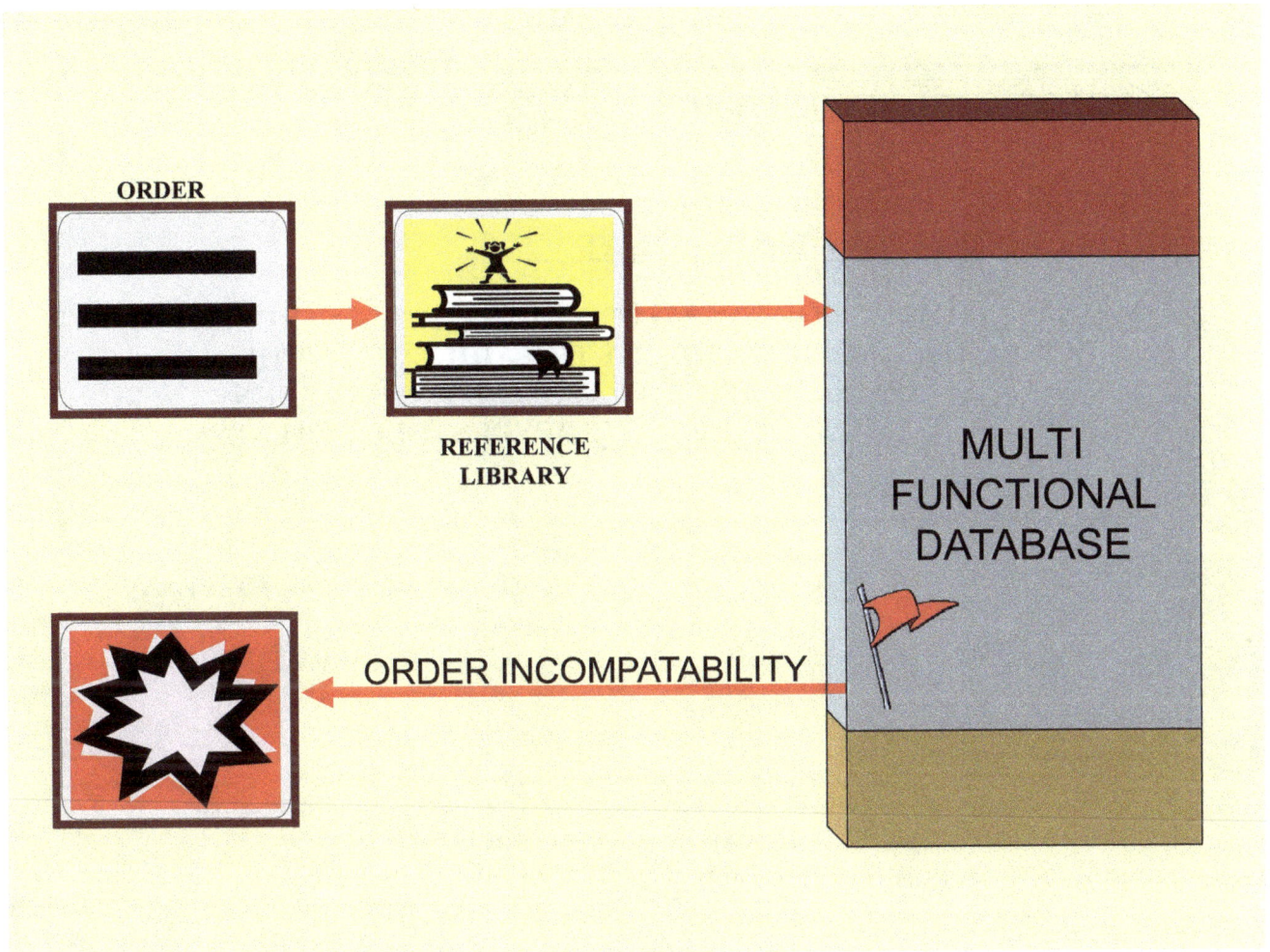

Incompatibility

The placing of this order automatically checks the database for any incompatibilities such as drug-to-drug, drug-to-lab, or other contra indicants, and will flag the physician regarding any such incompatibilities.

```
SMITH, SALLY   01-712-056-907


EDECRIN (ETHACRYNIC ACID)
TABLET ORAL-50 MG.-BID PC- 3 DAYS

MESSAGE:  THE USE OF KANAMYCIN SULFATE, (KANTREX) WITH
EDECRIN (ETHACRYNIC ACID), PARTICLARILY WHEN THE
DIURETIC IS ADMINISTERED INTRAVENIOUSLY, HAS BEEN
REPORTED TO CAUSE RAPID AND IRREVERSABLE DEAFNESS.

SELECT ONE OPTION:

CANCEL NEW ORDER                    EDUCATIONAL DISPLAY

CANCEL PREVIOUS ORDER               CONTINUE WITH ORDER
```

Active Keys	■ Exit	☐ Forward	☐ Print
	☐ Entry	■ Reverse	☐ Library

Cancels Previous Drug Order

The physician will automatically receive appropriate detailing or other library references, and they can either cancel or override such an alert … if deemed appropriate.

For Example: Here the database automatically notifies the physician that the patient is currently taking Kanamycin, which can cause irreversible deafness when taken with Edecrin. Therefore the physician cancels Kanamycin, to prevent such a drug-to-drug reaction.

```
 ┌──────────────────────────────────────────────────────────────┐
 │  SMITH, SALLY    01-712-056-907                               │
 │                                                              │
 │                                                              │
 │  EDECRIN (ETHACRYNIC ACID)                                   │
 │  TABLET ORAL-50 MG.-BID PC- 3 DAYS  FOR                      │
 │  PROB. #              NAME                    STATUS          │
 │        CODE               ONSET      ENTRY                   │
 │  # 01          CARDIOVASCULAR HEART FAILURE   ACTIVE         │
 │        270.0                  05/05          05/20           │
 │                                                              │
 │                                                              │
 │  CONFIRM                                    NOT CONFIRM      │
 │                                                              │
 └──────────────────────────────────────────────────────────────┘
```

| Active | ■ Exit | ☐ Forward | ☐ Print |
| Kcys | ☐ Entry | ■ Reverse | ☐ Library |

Confirms Order

The physician then confirms the order, sending the order to the database where it will notify the nursing station and the pharmacy to carry out that order. HSI found that even the most complex order took less than 10 selections to complete.

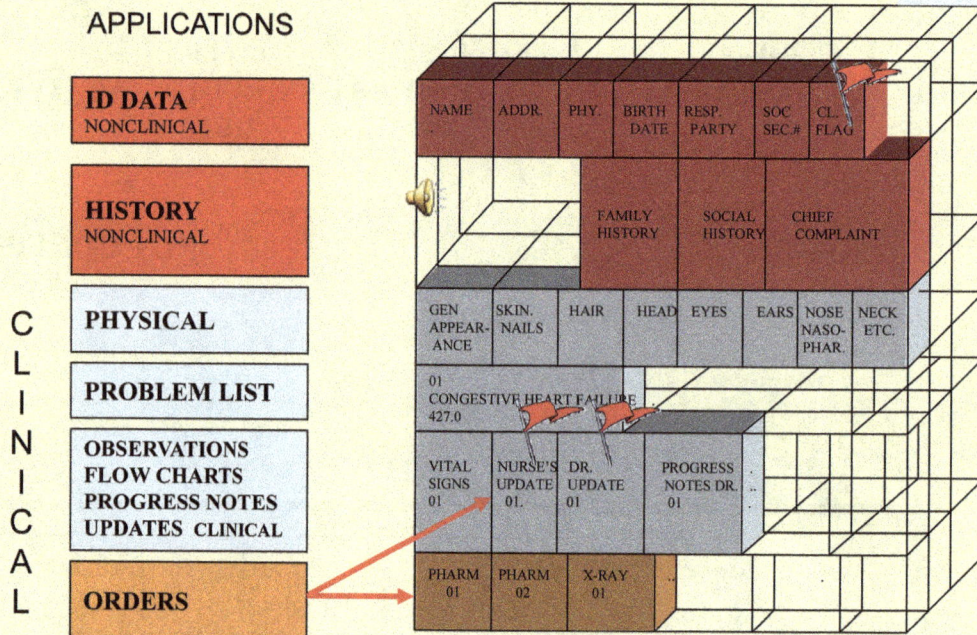

MULTIFUNCTIONAL HEALTHCARE DATABASE

Flag for Update Follow-Up

Entering all orders for prescriptions, examinations and treatments are usually made by problem or diagnosis, and the computer will automatically flag each order in the nurse and doctor's update until it is accomplished … monitoring any unreasonable time lapse between the order and the completion of the order.

```
 SMITH, SALLY    01-712-056-907



EDECRIN (ETHACRYNIC ACID)
TABLET ORAL-50 MG.-BID PC- 3 DAYS  FOR
PROB. #              NAME                        STATUS
        CODE              ONSET       ENTRY
# 01             CARDIOVASCULAR HEART FAILURE    ACTIVE
        270.0                  05/05        05/20




CONFIRM                                   NOT CONFIRM
```

Active	■ Exit	◻ Forward	◻ Print
Keys	◻ Entry	■ Reverse	◻ Library

Confirms Order

The physician then confirms the order, sending the order to the database where it will notify the nursing station and the pharmacy to carry out that order. HSI found that even the most complex order took less than 10 selections to complete.

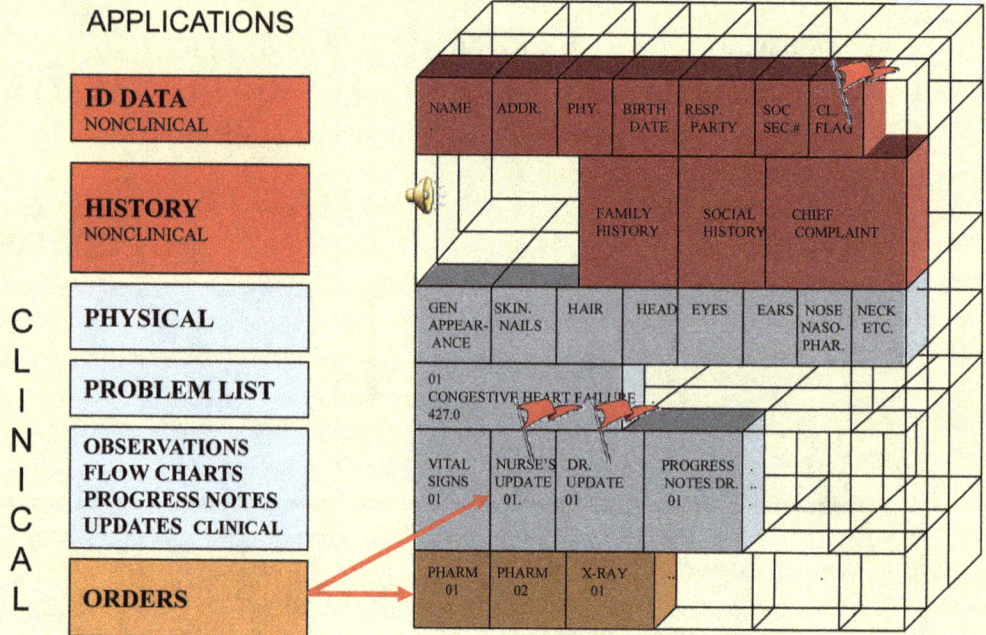

MULTIFUNCTIONAL HEALTHCARE DATABASE

Flag for Update Follow-Up

Entering all orders for prescriptions, examinations and treatments are usually made by problem or diagnosis, and the computer will automatically flag each order in the nurse and doctor's update until it is accomplished … monitoring any unreasonable time lapse between the order and the completion of the order.

```
SELECT ONE:


ENTER VITAL SIGNS                    ENTER PROGRESS NOTES

ENTER INTAKE/OUTPUT                  CONFIRM ROUTINE MEDS

ENTER PHYSICAL OBS.          ☞ ────  CONFIRM PRN STAT MEDS

ENTER EMOTIONAL OBS.                 CONFIRM TREATMENT ORDERS

ENTER ABNORMAL OBS.                  TYPE IN OBSERVATION
```

Active	■ Exit	☐ Forward	☐ Print
Keys	☐ Entry	■ Reverse	☐ Library

PRN-STAT Order

Once the nurse receives a medication order in the nursing update, they will go to their observation entry to confirm that they administered the medication in a timely manner. For example: Here a nurse elects to confirm a "PRN STAT" medication that was also ordered for Sally Smith.

```
CONFIRM PRN STAT MEDS:
Patient Name:  204-1 Smith, Sally Q.    # 01-712-056-907


  05/20/05 at 0900

  1415 LANOXIN (DIGOXIN)

  TABLET ORAL .75 MG STAT




CONFIRM                              NOT CONFIRM


  Active     ■ Exit      □ Forward    □ Print
  Keys       □ Entry     ■ Reverse    □ Library
```

Confirm Stat Order

As soon as the nurse confirms that this stat order was administered, the database will be updated. Most importantly, all completed orders will update accounts receivable, medical statistics, and more than one hundred sub-applications without any manual entry, eliminating almost all of the paper and most of the staff that currently do these chaotic tasks.

MULTIFUNCTIONAL HEALTHCARE DATABASE

APPLICATIONS

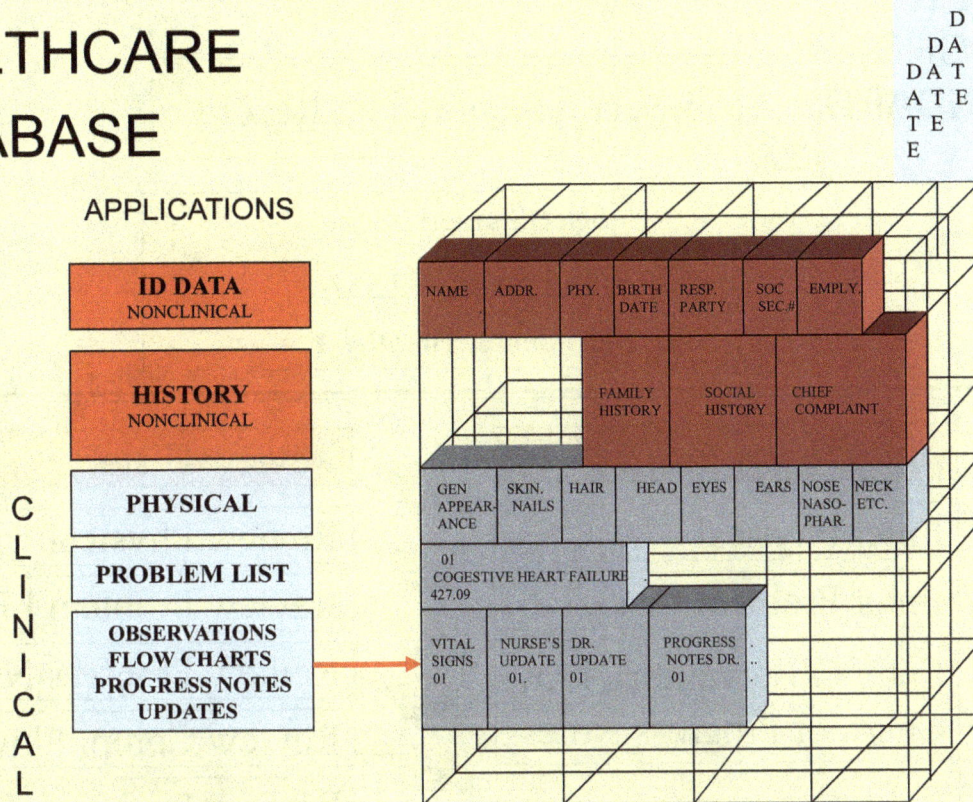

ID DATA NONCLINICAL	
HISTORY NONCLINICAL	
PHYSICAL	
PROBLEM LIST	
OBSERVATIONS FLOW CHARTS PROGRESS NOTES UPDATES	

C L I N I C A L

D D A T A D A T E T E E

NAME ADDR. PHY. BIRTH DATE RESP. PARTY SOC SEC.# EMPLY.

FAMILY HISTORY SOCIAL HISTORY CHIEF COMPLAINT

GEN APPEAR-ANCE SKIN. NAILS HAIR HEAD EYES EARS NOSE NASO-PHAR. NECK ETC.

01 COGESTIVE HEART FAILURE 427.09

VITAL SIGNS 01 NURSE'S UPDATE 01. DR. UPDATE 01 PROGRESS NOTES DR. 01

Observes Confirmation

After confirming the administration of this stat medication the computer removes the flags from database and notes that the medication was administered at 0900. If the appropriate confirmation is not accomplished within the designated time period, the problem can also be automatically referred for a later review or audit.

ACCESS HEALTH RECORD STANDARDS

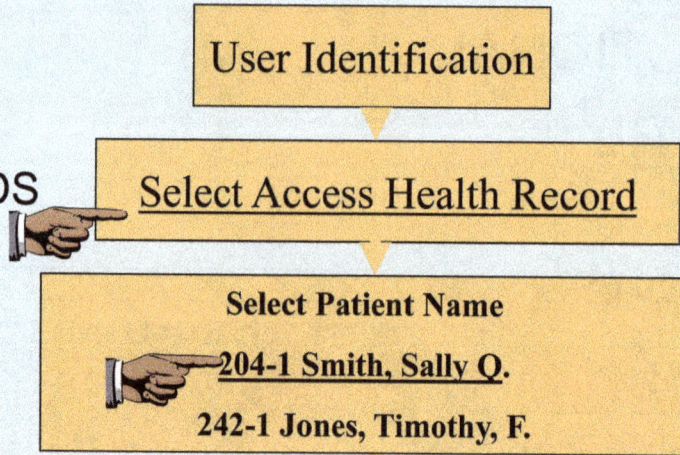

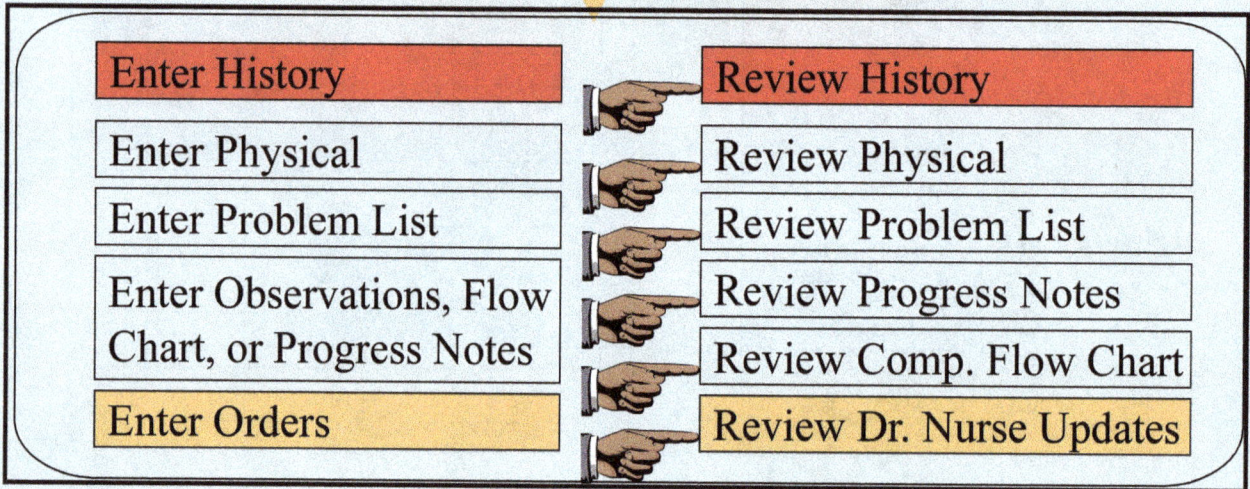

User Identification

Select Access Health Record

Select Patient Name

204-1 Smith, Sally Q.

242-1 Jones, Timothy, F.

Enter History	Review History
Enter Physical	Review Physical
Enter Problem List	Review Problem List
Enter Observations, Flow Chart, or Progress Notes	Review Progress Notes
	Review Comp. Flow Chart
Enter Orders	Review Dr. Nurse Updates

Review Applications

Whenever a qualified user wishes to review a patient's database, they can review the patient's history, physical, problem, progress note, comparative flow chart, or the physician or nurse's updates by just touching the appropriate category. Once they select an application, they can request all accumulative information under that category, all data by a specific date, all data by a specific problem ... such as Myocardial Infarction, or they can request any specific category within the medical record.

BY DATE 12/05/05

Select One:

PREVIUOS MEDICAL HISTORY

FAMILY HISTORY

SOCIAL HISTORY

CHIEF COMPLAINT

MULTIFUNCTIONAL HEALTHCARE DATABASE

DDATE

APPLICATIONS

ID DATA
NONCLINICAL

HISTORY
NONCLINICAL

PHYSICAL

PROBLEM LIST

OBSERVATIONS
FLOW CHARTS
PROGRESS NOTES
UPDATES CLINICAL

ORDERS

CLINICAL

NAME	ADDR.	PHY.	BIRTH DATE	RESP. PARTY	SOC SEC.#	EMPLY.	ETC
PREVIOUS MEDICAL HISTORY		FAMILY HISTORY		SOCIAL HISTORY		CHIEF COMPLAINT	12/05/05
GEN APPEAR-ANCE	SKIN. NAILS	HAIR	HEAD	EYES	EARS	NOSE NASO-PHAR.	NECK ETC.
01 CONGESTIVE HEART FAILURE 410.9			02 RHEUMATIC FEVER ACTIVE PERICARDITIS			ETC.	
VITAL SIGNS 01	NURSE'S UPDATE 01.	DR. UPDATE 01		PROGRESS NOTES DR. 01	NURSING OBSERV... 02	DR. OBSERV... 01 ETC.	
PHARM 01	PHARM 02	X-RAY 01	LAB.. 01		P.T 02	DIET. O1 ETC.	

Review by Date

The patient's multifunctional database can call out specific information by date, such as the history that was recorded on 12/05/05. They could also call out the most current history, the previous medical history, family history, social history, or chief complaint by date. Physical exams, problems or diagnoses, observations, orders, and ID can all be obtained by the date entered.

BY ACCUMULATIVE
PHYSICAL EXAM DATA
Doe, John   10/03/02 TO 12/10/05
SELECT ONE:
GENERAL APPEARANCE   EYES
SKIN NAILS   EARS
HAIR   NOSE
HEAD   NECK ETC.

MULTIFUNCTIONAL
HEALTHCARE
DATABASE

APPLICATIONS

ID DATA
NONCLINICAL

HISTORY
NONCLINICAL

PHYSICAL

PROBLEM LIST

OBSERVATIONS
FLOW CHARTS
PROGRESS NOTES
UPDATES CLINICAL

ORDERS

C L I N I C A L

| NAME | ADDR. | PHY. | BIRTH DATE | RESP. PARTY | SOC SEC.# | EMPLY. | ETC |

| PREVIOUS MEDICAL HISTORY | FAMILY HISTORY | SOCIAL HISTORY | CHIEF COMPLAINT |

| GEN APPEAR-ANCE | SKIN. NAILS | HAIR | HEAD | EYES | EARS | NOSE NASO-PHAR. | NECK ETC. |

| CONGESTIVE HEART FAILURE 427.0 | RHEUMATIC FEVER ACTIVE PERICARDITIS | ETC. |

| VITAL SIGNS 01 | NURSE'S UPDATE 01. | DR. UPDATE 01 | PROGRESS NOTES DR. 01 | NURSING OBSERV... 02 | DR. OBSERV.. 01 ETC. |

| PHARM 01 | PHARM 02 | X-RAY 01 | LAB.. 01 | P.T 02 | DIET. 01 ETC. |

Review Accumulative Data

The patient's multifunctional database can also call out all accumulative physical exam information stored in the database, as well as all accumulative ID, history, problem, or all observations and order information.

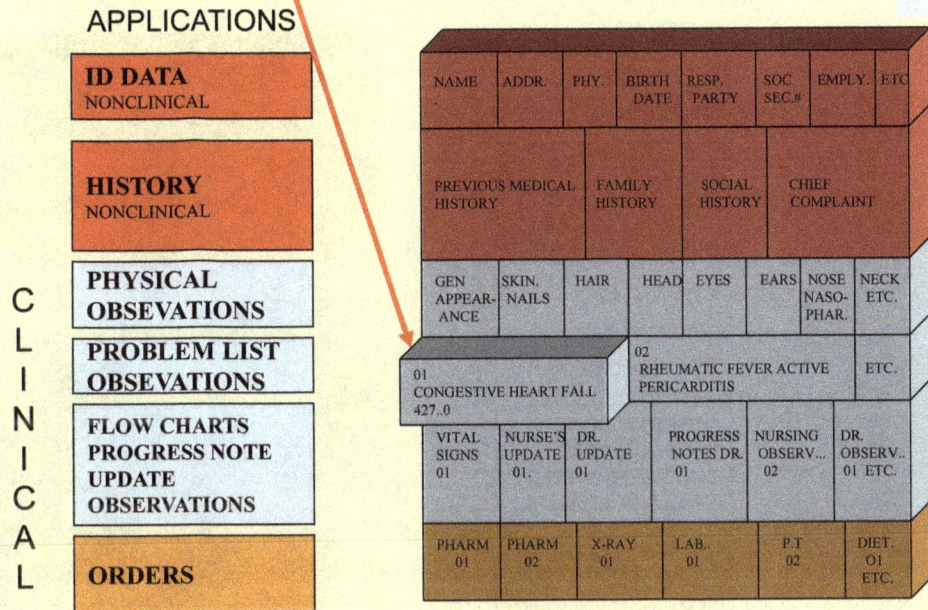

BY PROBLEM

Doe, John

Problem #, Name, Status
Code, Reference, Onset Date, Entry Date
1 Congestive Heart Failure
427.0 01 01 05 01 20 A

MULTIFUNCTIONAL HEALTHCARE DATABASE

DATE DATE

APPLICATIONS

CLINICAL

ID DATA
NONCLINICAL

HISTORY
NONCLINICAL

PHYSICAL
OBSEVATIONS

PROBLEM LIST
OBSEVATIONS

FLOW CHARTS
PROGRESS NOTE
UPDATE
OBSERVATIONS

ORDERS

NAME | ADDR. | PHY. | BIRTH DATE | RESP. PARTY | SOC SEC.# | EMPLY. | ETC

PREVIOUS MEDICAL HISTORY | FAMILY HISTORY | SOCIAL HISTORY | CHIEF COMPLAINT

GEN APPEAR-ANCE | SKIN. NAILS | HAIR | HEAD | EYES | EARS | NOSE NASO-PHAR. | NECK ETC.

01 CONGESTIVE HEART FALL 427..0 | 02 RHEUMATIC FEVER ACTIVE PERICARDITIS | ETC.

VITAL SIGNS 01 | NURSE'S UPDATE 01. | DR. UPDATE 01 | PROGRESS NOTES DR. 01 | NURSING OBSERV... 02 | DR. OBSERV... 01 ETC.

PHARM 01 | PHARM 02 | X-RAY 01 | LAB. 01 | P.T 02 | DIET. O1 ETC.

Review Data by Problem

The multifunctional database can also review a patient's specific problem, symptom, diagnosis, or sub diagnosis ... their physical by problem ... as well as all orders, observations, flow charts, progress notes and updates by problem. Statistics and treatment results for committee review can also be analyzed and audited by problem or diagnostic code, without ever seeing the patient's name, unless required.

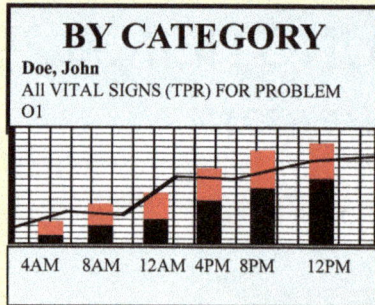

Review Data by Category

The user can also dynamically request data by category, such as all vital sign, which can then be displayed on either a graphical flow chart or bar graph. The dynamic tailoring of one's own specific categories, offers great potential for the team management of a patient's treatment in the future.

SOURCE DATA
SUB-APPLICATIONS (OVER 100)

I. SOURCE DATA
A. Registration
  1. Admission List
    Inpatient
    Outpatient
  2. Census
    Station
    Total
    Accumulative
  3. Transfer List
    Physician
    Patient
    Administrative
  4. Discharge List
    Inpatient
    Outpatient
  5. Scheduling
    Inpatient
    Outpatient
B. Master Population File
C. Medical Statistical System
  1. Disease Index
  2. Operative Index
  3. Physician's Index
  4. Patient Service Statistics

II. ADMINISTRATIVE
A. Administrative
  1. Policy
  2. General Objectives
  3. Departmental Objectives
  4. Public Relations
  5. Administrative Reports and Statistics
  6. Financial Budgeting
  7. Physician's Files
B. Business Office
  1. General Journal Accounting
    Financial Reports
  2. Accounts Receivable
  3. Accounts Payable
  4. Payroll

C. Materials Management
  1. Purchasing
    General
    Departmental (Dietary, Pharmaceutical)
    Product Analysis, Standardization
  2. Inventory
    General
    Departmental
    Central Supply
D. General Services
  1. Housekeeping
    Bed Preparation
    General
  2. Laundry
    Patient, Station, and Department
    General
  3. Maintenance
    Preventive
    General
  4. Engineering
    Preventive
    General
E. Personnel
  1. Recruiting, Screening and Hiring
  2. Health Services
  3. Staffing (General and Departmental)
    Manning Tables
    Scheduling
  4. Position Control
    (Personnel Budgeting)
  5. Termination Processing
  6. Wage and Salary
    Point Curve
  7. Employee Policy
    Contracts
  8. Procedures

  9. Job Descriptions
    Point System
  10. Job Analysis
  11. Employee Relations
  12. In-service Education
    Orientation- Employees
    Orientation-Professional
    Formal Education-Employees
    Patient Education
    General
    Clinical
F. Communications
  1. Messenger Service
  2. Internal
  3. External

III. ANCILLARY SERVICES
A. Laboratory-Exam and Test Libraries- Update Reports and department system
B. Pharmacy-Formulary Library and Updates
C. Cardio Pulmonary, EKG, Pulmonary Function and Shock Monitoring Libraries and Updates
D. Dietary Menu's Library, Food Production, Recipes, and Dietetics
E. Radiology- Exam and Test Libraries, Updates and Department System
F. Social Service- Internal, External and Department Systems
G. Physical Therapy-Treatment Library, Updates, and Department System
H. Occupational Therapy- Treatment Library (Therapeutic and Diversional) –Updates and Department System
I. Electroenchepalography-Treatment Library, Updates, and Department System

Sub-Applications

Over one hundred sub applications can be integrated with source data with almost no manual entry, and it's been estimated that a comprehensive communications system would not only improve the quality of care, but could cut costs by as much as 50% if health professionals could once again be persuaded to work together toward a national master plan based on professional standards.

TODAY'S MEDICAL RECORDS

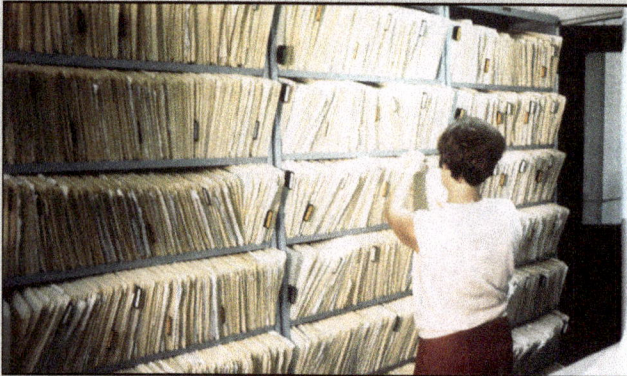

HEALTHCARE FORMS

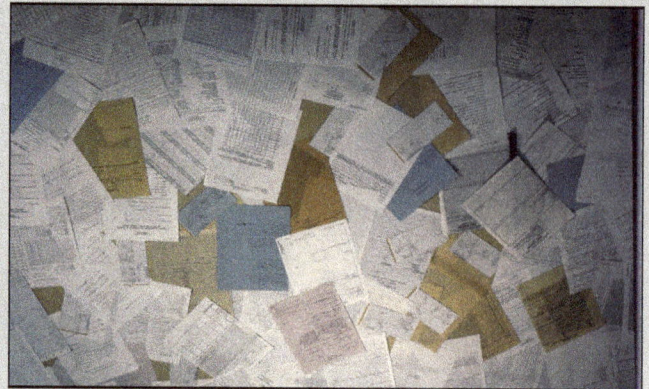

Today's Medical Record Files & Today's Paper Forms

Patient information has been stored in hundreds of decentralized files such as these. Expensive Staff are required to prepare and maintain these costly and chaotic paper systems that duplicate patient information over and over and then store them in what is often an irretrievable manner ... creating decentralized systems that defy any comprehensive overview of the patient's wellbeing.

HSI found that the average hospital has some 360 forms they continually hand carry from one location to another, each requiring costly preparation and duplication of much of the same information over and over. This huge pile of paper eventually comes to rest where it's seldom readily available. Some of the hospital's HSI studied had as many as 16 hundred forms. Previous studies indicated the average form cost was a dollar twenty seven cents, ignoring the cost of the messenger systems and the traffic filled corridors. As a result, mistakes are made, and information is overlooked as patients fall victim to all this chaos.

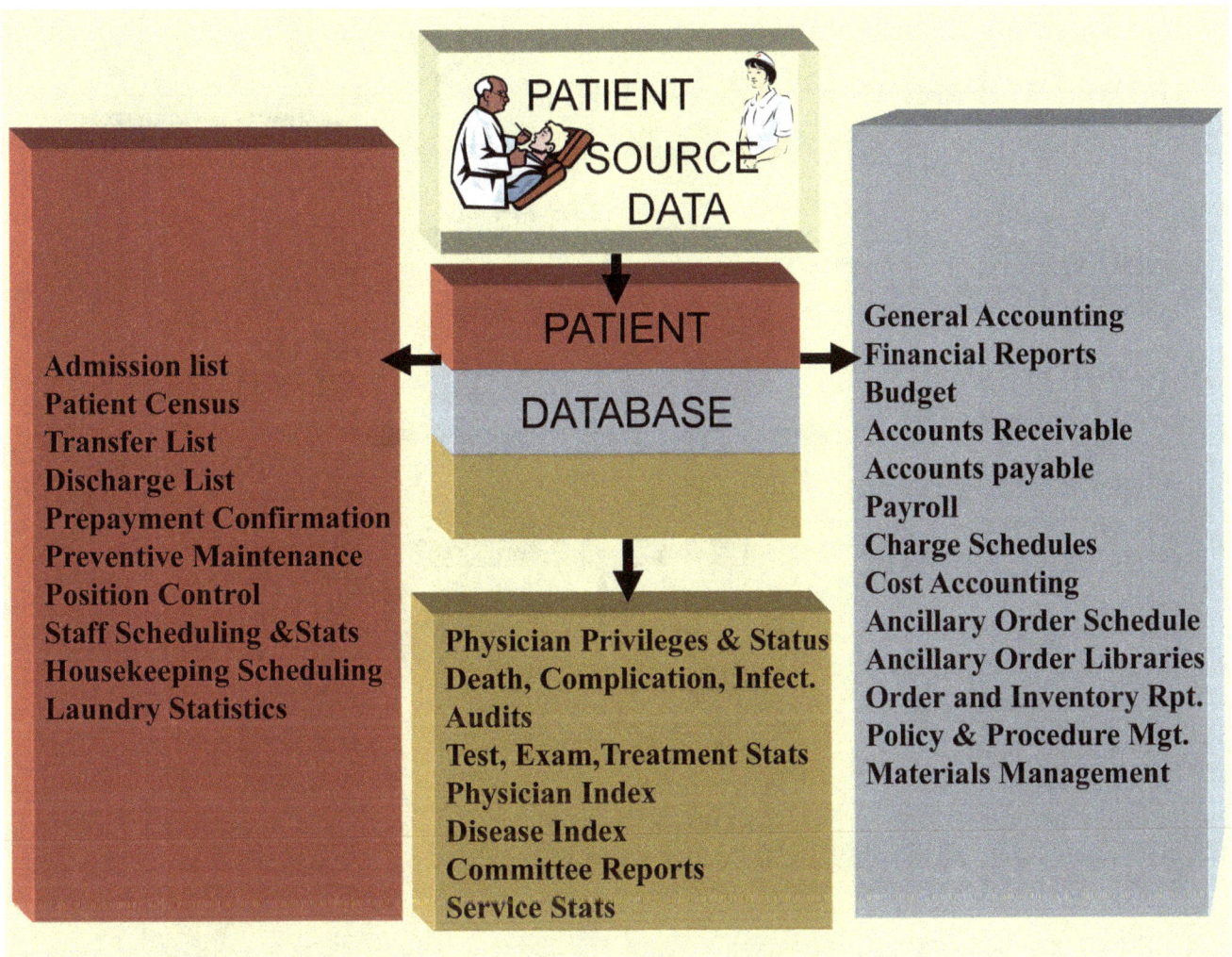

PATIENT SOURCE DATA

PATIENT DATABASE

Admission list
Patient Census
Transfer List
Discharge List
Prepayment Confirmation
Preventive Maintenance
Position Control
Staff Scheduling &Stats
Housekeeping Scheduling
Laundry Statistics

Physician Privileges & Status
Death, Complication, Infect.
Audits
Test, Exam,Treatment Stats
Physician Index
Disease Index
Committee Reports
Service Stats

General Accounting
Financial Reports
Budget
Accounts Receivable
Accounts payable
Payroll
Charge Schedules
Cost Accounting
Ancillary Order Schedule
Ancillary Order Libraries
Order and Inventory Rpt.
Policy & Procedure Mgt.
Materials Management

Manual Reports

Here are just a few of today's many manual reports that will require almost no manual preparation in the future. For example: Patient's charges can be automatically applied when a nurse confirms a lab test, an x-ray, or when a drug has been given — totally automating accounts receivable. Once a piece of equipment is used to treat a patient a predefined number of times, a preventive maintenance work sheet can be automatically prepared for that piece of equipment. Admissions, deaths, complications and infections can all be accurately prepared without departments tediously finding, reviewing and recording this information manually. Nameless treatment statistics can be automatically prepared for monthly service and audit reports and on and on.

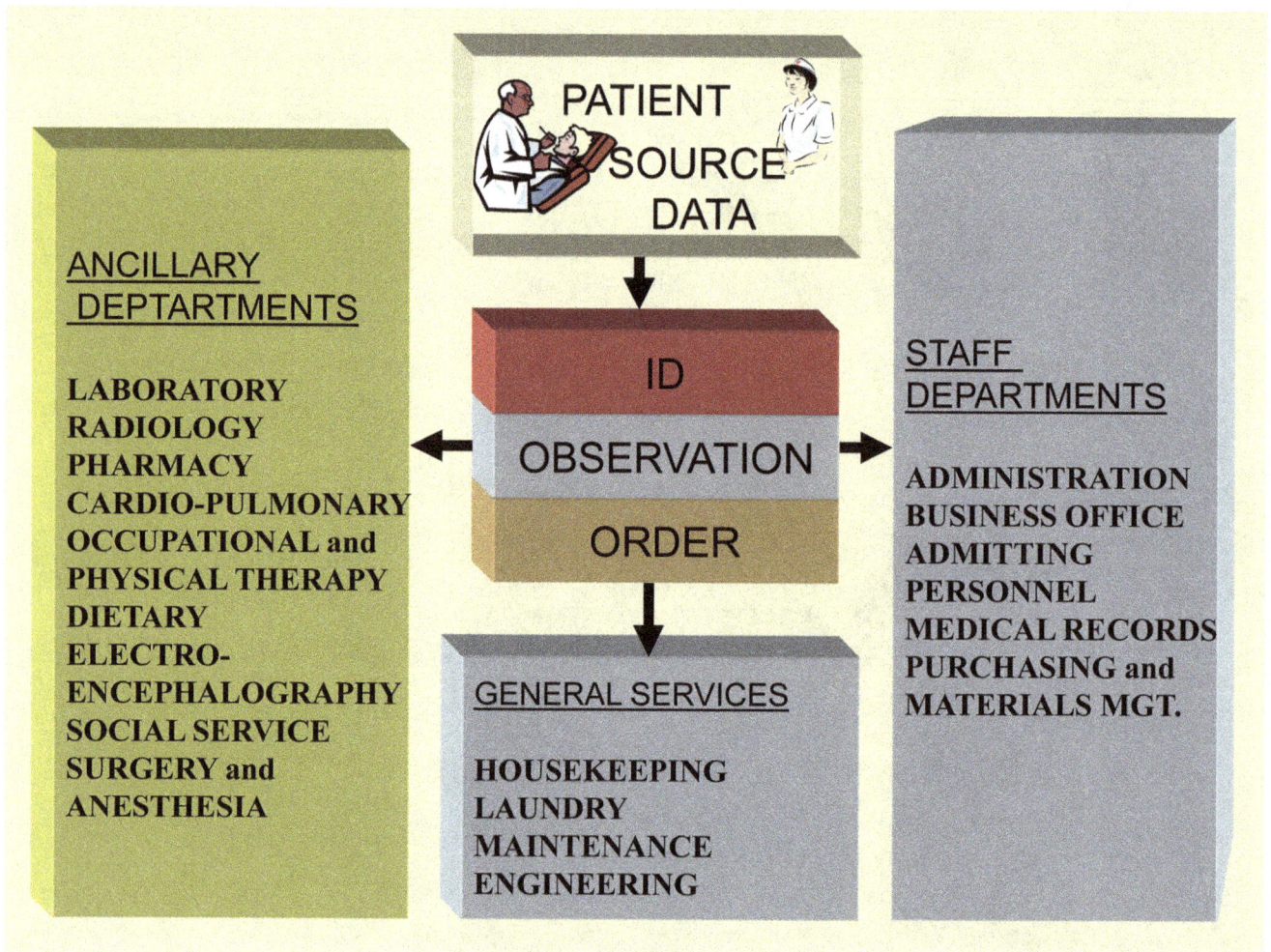

ANCILLARY DEPTARTMENTS

LABORATORY
RADIOLOGY
PHARMACY
CARDIO-PULMONARY
OCCUPATIONAL and
PHYSICAL THERAPY
DIETARY
ELECTRO-ENCEPHALOGRAPHY
SOCIAL SERVICE
SURGERY and ANESTHESIA

PATIENT SOURCE DATA

ID

OBSERVATION

ORDER

STAFF DEPARTMENTS

ADMINISTRATION
BUSINESS OFFICE
ADMITTING
PERSONNEL
MEDICAL RECORDS
PURCHASING and MATERIALS MGT.

GENERAL SERVICES

HOUSEKEEPING
LAUNDRY
MAINTENANCE
ENGINEERING

Source Point

Capturing patient information where it first occurs, at source point, helps eliminate errors and the costly re-entry of confidential patient information over and over. This can and should be accomplished in every healthcare facility at the local, state, or national level under a single comprehensive system for every citizen of the United States. When a patient first registers into the future single health care system, or a qualified health professional places an order or records a patient observation, confidentiality and clinical ethics standards must be assured equally for every citizen regardless of age, sex, service, job, or where one lives.

DESIGN STANDARDS
for a
HEALTH RECORD
DATABASE NETWORK ©

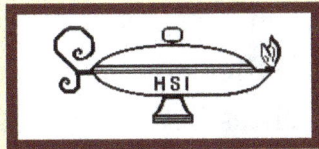

By
HEALTH SYSTEMS INSTITUTE

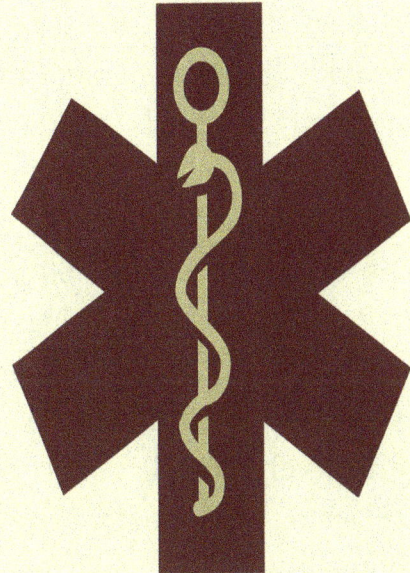

Summary

Before the twentieth-century, untrained charlatans practiced medicine that was traced back to the Witch-Doctors who attempted to cure sickness and exorcise evil spirits through witchcraft, magic, and secret rituals. This Witch Doctor Syndrome conditioned the untrained healthcare practitioners in the early twentieth-century to acquire knowledge to gain prestige and control over a totally disorganized and decentralized art form that intentionally resisted the development of any standards, rules, regulations, and laws. That was until educational standards were clearly defined in the 1910 *"Flexner Report"* by the Carnegie and Rockefeller Foundations, which pointed up many serious conditions that were *scandalous*. This report proposed that patients should receive care from properly trained physicians and it established medical education standards and the licensing of trained and qualified physicians that took the *"Hippocratic Oath"* of *"Do No Harm."* However, today's spiraling healthcare costs are clearly harming those sick and disabled that cannot afford to obtain proper health care. In an attempt to solve this problem, Blue Cross was founded in 1929, and Blue Shield in 1939, which formed Blue Cross and Blue Shield (BCBS), which became a very successful ***privately owned nonprofit-noninsurance pre-payment program*** that paid no taxes and was regulated by each state as a ***Community Rated System*** — meaning everyone paid the same rate, regardless of age, sex, where he or she lived, or how sick they were. Then in 1946, the Hill-Burton Hospital Survey and Construction Act helped nonprofit hospitals by providing federal grants that guaranteed loans to improve this country's nonprofit hospitals, which became the first government program formed to help meet the hospital growth needs required to treat all the injured veterans from two world wars. The government also used tax dollars to accomplish a 4.5-bed ratio per a 1,000 population for these nonprofit hospitals that were not allowed to discriminate based on race, color, national origin, or creed, while providing a reasonable amount of uncompensated care for twenty years. At that time, tax dollars were efficiently managed very cost effectively for all nonprofit programs such as healthcare, education, and selected infrastructure projects, which were then designed to benefit humanity as a whole. Then in 1945, Congress, in direct opposition to these nonprofit services to humanity, shockingly passed the McCarran-Ferguson Act. This Act ushered competitive profit-seeking insurance companies into this country's healthcare system, which increased healthcare costs dramatically by adding a profit to the cost of healthcare, and in so doing, the United States became the only country in the world to seek profit from their sick and disabled. In an attempt to conceal the McCarran-Ferguson mistake – Congress in 1965 passed Medicare and Medicaid where Medicare provided health care coverage for those who are 65 or older or had a severe disability, and Medicaid became a state and federal program that provides health coverage for those with a very low income. Congress also chose to once again partner with BCBS to administer Medicare, while secretly creating a special government healthcare insurance program for themselves. Then in the mid 60's, profit insurance and the pharmaceutical industry aggressively lobbied Congress with favors and the cost for these political donations were placed directly on the backs of our sick and disabled. With fewer patients being able to afford healthcare, our world healthcare ranking dropped from first to thirty-second as ranked by the World Health Organization (WHO). Then in the late 1960's, profit insurance aggressively moved to take over this country's health care prepayment system, by forcefully pursuing only the healthy clients and working groups to buy cheaper **tiered** low-risk **group rated** profit insurance—knowing full well that these clients did not have a clue that each group rate would significantly increase as its members decreased in number due to health related problems and age. This forced the Blues to cover more of the aged, sick and disabled, and pregnancies, which profit insurance dumped by increasing these patient's premiums to unrealistic levels. And since healthcare was not receiving any trickledown profits from profit insurance to improve patient care, hospitals began to experience huge financial losses as insurance profits began to spiral healthcare costs out of control. As a result, hospitals across the country were forced to develop Regional Planning and Cost Containment Programs, and in 1962, this author was persuaded to incorporate Health Systems Institute (HSI) and serve as the President and Principle Investigator to study computer applications for hospitals while continuing to manage hospitals. Later, in 1979, as the Chairperson of a Regional Cost Containment Committee, this author spent a full day with Gerald Ford, the former President of the United States, seeking his advice on how healthcare might return to a single nonprofit prepayment system. After that meeting, Gerald Ford put his arm over John's shoulder and said: "John, the healthcare system will have to collapse before things get better." Although this author did not believe him then, he does now, and that's why he decided to publish HSI's "Conceptual Design Standards," which proposes a single nonprofit health record communications network that will help Americans to understand and support the enormous job that is going to be every bit as big as the U.S. space program. This HSI research placed more than a thousand voluntary doctors, nurses, and paraprofessionals and the Universities of Michigan State, Minnesota, Michigan, Iowa, and the Charles T. Miller Hospital in St. Paul, MN and the St Lawrence Hospital in Lansing, MI on committees to assist with the design and development of a single computer based medical record. HSI studies initially determined that the average hospital paper medical record usually comprised more than 375 separate and distinct medical record paper forms. Not only was it very costly to create this variety of forms in a hospital, but it's even more expensive to move all this paper manually into a system that is totally decentralized, and not very confidential or legally protected. A single comprehensive on-line computer based network of patient owned health records offers the only solution to today's decentralized paper chaos – and since the primary ownership and legal rights to a patient's medical record actually does rest with the patient, this nation needs to stop creating these decentralized manual medical records that are currently not readily available to the patient because they are stored in this confusing maze of decentralized multiple healthcare facilities, and it's only getting worse — which inherently denies patient responsibility. Perhaps it's more comfortable for patients to not be responsible for their own bad habits involving diets, smoking, alcohol, drugs, sexual behavior, or maintaining one's own physical or mental well-being. However, it's absolutely necessary for the patient or their designate to assume greater responsibility for one's own well-being, and to do this the patient needs to maintain legal ownership of a well-defined single computer based medical record so they can have immediate access to their total clinical information. The patient or their designate should also be responsible for maintaining and updating their own personal information as well as efficiently control the release of selected clinical information to the appropriate healthcare professional or facility on a strictly confidential basis from either their own personal computer, or when they seek service from any of the system's authorized on-line locations. When authorized by the patient or their designate, the selected on-line facility or professional individual should have access only to the required legally protected confidential database to review and/or update the patient's clinical information. However, security to this single system must be accurately defined, approved, and maintained before this comprehensive universal cost effective system is allowed to become functional. Many thought that flying to the moon was impossible, and HSI has proven that a single patient record is not only possible but essential — and it should also be understood that this is a huge undertaking that is every bit as big as the space shots this nation has already accomplished successfully, which will also require government financial support. Years of HSI evaluating and defining these future concepts have confirmed that the consumer will also someday demand and understand the importance of these required major changes and improvements in order to stop the unmanageable and non-confidential chaos that currently is tolerated by so many trusting patients. A patient database will not only advance and significantly improve patient treatment, but it will put a stop to the current misuse of patient information. Although such a system will be very costly up front, it will eventually cut healthcare costs dramatically when fully implemented. Projections by HSI have determined this could realistically cut healthcare costs by as much as fifty-percent, however, this type of system can only be developed if highly skilled healthcare professionals are allowed to assume total responsibility, which excludes uninformed politicians and corporate profit seekers from ever again taking over total control of this highly professional and technical human service. A legally confidential universal database will also, for the first time, permit critical analysis, evaluation, and measurement of the quality of patient care without ever exposing the patient's or doctor's identity unless it necessarily becomes required. Some of today's computer system have helped the patient to better communicate with the doctor by reviewing reports and scheduling appointments and ordering drugs, but now healthcare professionals have to design and develop a legally confidential database that will also allow the consumers to measure and audit overall medical staff performance accurately and confidentially. Hospitals currently conduct manual medical record audits by patient name and these non-comprehensive audits are too often accomplished by one's close physician's peers, who are too closely associated with the physician being audited. Audit of a physician by their close associates can constitute a conflict of interest, but only professionally trained physicians can develop such a tool that can automatically set basic clinical standards that help regulate, monitor, audit, advise and suggest alternatives in making and assisting with the individual judgment and evaluation of every clinical practice. Because the average physician initially suspects the computer is a policing tool, they sometimes have difficulty in accepting the computer as a supportive tool that can significantly benefit the total practice of medicine — however, there is a growing number of physicians that are now recognizing and supporting the wisdom of a paperless record if they are allowed to set the standards. Malpractice, injury, improper treatment, unnecessary tests and poor patient care can be reduced meaningfully by providing an adequate patient database if doctors are allowed to provide the necessary leadership and cooperatively help in designing such a tool that will benefit healthcare and not depend on today's unskilled profit centered programmers or nonclinical insurance executives.

Today's manual health record usually includes a medical record face sheet that records patient identifying information, with a summary of the admitting diagnosis or problem, the final diagnosis, and the principal procedures which are manually coded, each with an interpretable number.

Laboratory, radiology, pharmacy, dietary, physical therapy, occupational therapy, cardiology, encephalography and numerous other ancillary service reports are currently filed separately and not integrated with the diagnosis into a comprehensive, multi-facility patient health record database. Today's hospital or clinic's manual records are also filed under a terminal-digit numbering system, which permits an individual patient's record to be filed only within that facilities individual numbering system. A codified, comprehensive, cumulative, interpretable, family unit number for multiple facilities has yet to be defined. HSI developed such a family and genetic coding, and this will be a very important factor in the future of preventive medicine. In 1967, HSI hired a staff of temporary clerical employees to accomplish the enormous job of re-numbering every patient's manual medical record at the St. Lawrence Hospital under a family unit numbering system. Anticipating that the human genome map will soon decipher the chemical book of life for the human organism, identifying highly confidential patient and family heredity characteristics and DNA data will play a major part in healthcare, which requires creating a family unit database. Standard diagnostic workups, with a problem and symptom library that directs or guides the physician to a list of prospective diagnoses or differential diagnoses, are absent in today's manual patient's medical record and an automatic coding of diagnoses and procedures has yet to be implemented. Because of this, orders for a diagnostic workup or the treatment of a defined diagnosis cannot be dynamically monitored to determine either the treatment regimen or its success ratio. Accurate, dynamic computer-based health record statistics on treatment procedures, diseases, deaths, complications, infections, function, etiology, topography, or heredity, by geographic location, are yet to be dynamically implemented and made available for comprehensive patient care, education, audit, or planning. Setting scientific standards for the practice of medicine does not necessitate a rigid non-innovative system, but rather one that allows flexibility as it reasonably monitors and measures variations in medical practice. Accurate patient database statistics will be essential if health education and preventive care are ever to be effectively advanced. It is embarrassing to find that America's automobile manufacturers, electricians, and plumbers currently have better standards for consumer protection than healthcare in the United States. Patient database tools and diagnostic assistance are long overdue in today's non-system, which far too often professes to provide the best health care in the world, yet is currently ranked 32nd in the world. National greatness can only be measured by the quality of this nation's advancements.